The Pregnancy Diet

*A Healthy Weight Control Program
for Pregnant Women*

Eileen Behan, R.D.

POCKET BOOKS
New York   London   Toronto   Sydney   Tokyo   Singapore

An *Original* Publication of POCKET BOOKS

POCKET BOOKS, a division of Simon & Schuster Inc.
1230 Avenue of the Americas, New York, NY 10020

Library of Congress Cataloging-in-Publication Data

Behan, Eileen.
    The pregnancy diet : a healthy weight control program for pregnant women / Eileen Behan.
        p.   cm.
    Includes bibliographical references and index.
    ISBN 0-671-00393-3
    1. Pregnancy—Nutritional aspects—Popular works. 2. Mothers— Nutrition—Popular works. 3. Prenatal care—Popular works. I. Title.
RG559.B44   1999
618.2′4—dc21   98-53461

First Pocket Books trade paperback printing January 1999

10 9 8 7 6 5 4 3 2 1

Cover design by Rod Hernandez, front cover photo © David A. Wagner/Phototake/PNI
Book design by Nancy Singer

Printed in the U.S.A.

FEEL CONFIDENT ABOUT FOOD AGAIN!
DO YOU KNOW . . .

- how many calories you should have every day to gain just the right amount for you *and your baby?*
- how to control cravings (or should you just eat what you desire)?
- how your metabolism will change during and after pregnancy?
- whether breast-feeding helps you lose weight?
- what foods you should eat—and what you should avoid?
- the stunning truth about pregnancy, weight, and postpartum weight loss?
- what to do if you're overweight when you become pregnant? What if you're underweight?
- what really makes women gain too much weight during pregnancy?
- *and* that you can indulge in Chocolate Bread Pudding with Meringue, Baked Macaroni and Cheese, a Breakfast Burrito, or Very Vegetable Soup (with Cheese)—and still gain just the right amount? (Yes, you can!)

GET ALL THE REASSURING ANSWERS IN
THE PREGNANCY DIET

Also by Eileen Behan

Microwave Cooking for Your Baby and Child
Eat Well, Lose Weight While Breastfeeding
Meals that Heal for Babies, Toddlers, and Children*

Available from Pocket Books

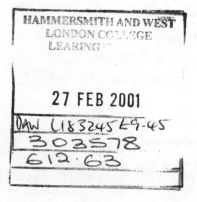
For orders other than by individual consumers, Pocket Books grants a discount on the purchase of **10 or more** copies of single titles for special markets or premium use. For further details, please write to the Vice-President of Special Markets, Pocket Books, 1633 Broadway, New York, NY 10019-6785, 8th Floor.

For information on how individual consumers can place orders, please write to Mail Order Department, Simon & Schuster Inc., 200 Old Tappan Road, Old Tappan, NJ 07675.

Lovingly dedicated to my mother, Elizabeth Behan, who shared her love of cooking and much more; to David, who always supports me; and to Sarah and Emily, who make life much more interesting.

Acknowledgments

Sharon and Sheila, thanks for being sisters who are encouraging and supportive. Trish Cronan and Brad Lavigne, thank you for your enthusiasm for life and being the kind of friends who are always available when really needed. Judy Paige, you have been a help to me as a writer and nutritionist, but even more so as my very dear friend. Madeleine Walsh, thank you for taking the time to read part of this manuscript, and Marilyn DeSimone, I always appreciate your frank comments on life and work. Jennifer Quirk, thank you for sharing your expertise on exercise and pregnancy.

Sally Ann Lederman, Ph.D., thank you for your review and comments on parts of this manuscript. Your input made for a clearer and more accurate final product. Casey Bloomer, R.N.P., thank you for your comments about the medical complications covered in this book. Sarah MacDuffie, D.O., thank you for sharing your medical expertise and finding time to read the manuscript. At Pocket Books I would like to thank Emily Bestler, a superb and enthusiastic editor, and Jill Hasty and Lauren Rott, who make the publishing process run smoothly. Special thanks to Carol Mann.

Contents

Introduction

In our culture, there is a great premium placed on being thin. For many women it is a lifetime goal, a cherished ideal. There have even been surveys that found that some respondents would give up five years of life if they could be thin. Pregnancy is the one time we are expected, even encouraged, to gain weight. It is the speed bump on the diet highway of life. When I was pregnant with my second child, ten months after my first (and five pounds away from my goal weight), I was actually relieved to be pregnant again because it meant I could gain weight and not worry about the approaching bathing suit season. But for other women pregnancy can be a great cause of anxiety if they fear the weight gain recommended by their doctor.

One survey discovered that as many as 40 percent of first-time mothers worry that they will gain too much weight while pregnant, and 72 percent fear they will be unable to return to their former weight. In another study, 100 women interviewed about their weight three days after giving birth reported that they made a conscious effort to "watch their weight" while pregnant. The alarming news was that some of these women chose cigarette smoking and induced vomiting as means of weight control.

While it is appropriate to be concerned about nutrition while pregnant, it is not okay or even accurate to fear a permanent weight gain caused by pregnancy alone. Many women I have counselled about nutrition have identified pregnancy as the cause of their weight gain. When I began research on the relationship between obesity and pregnancy I expected to find a rock-solid connection between the two. Instead I found that most women who gain the recommended amounts while pregnant retain only two to three pounds, 6 to 12 months after delivery.

Women who have a strong fear of gaining weight may not gain the weight they need, and this can translate into poor nutrition for the mother and a low birth weight for the baby. On the other hand, excessive weight gain carries health risks to mother and child as well. The mother who gains significantly above the recommended weight guidelines can increase both her risk of medical complications at delivery and her risk for obesity. The research does suggest that women who gain above the recommended weight ranges will retain more weight 12 months after delivery.

Permanent weight gain is not a trivial health issue: One-third of American adults are now overweight, up from one-quarter a decade ago. Women who are very overweight have a much greater risk of heart disease, up to three times that of women who are not as heavy. But the research does not identify pregnancy as the cause of permanent weight gain. Instead, the rise in weight gain is more the result of inactivity, too much food, and very often a change in lifestyle brought on by motherhood.

Weight is very important during pregnancy. Too little suggests poor nutrition, but too much increases the risk of medical complications. Neither situation is acceptable. The ideal is to find the middle ground, to eat a diet that keeps your body healthy and your baby developing at its very best. No one can predict with certainty exactly how your body will gain weight while you are pregnant. Most doctors will recommend a gain of 25 to 35 pounds. Some women will be advised to gain more, some less, depending on weight, height, and age. You cannot really control weight gain, you can only control what you choose to eat and the exercise you do.

Women are advised not to diet while pregnant, and all reasonable women already know that weight gain comes with pregnancy. What women seem to need are realistic guidelines about how much weight to gain and how fast. Most important, they need recommendations on what to do when weight gain is excessive or inadequate. "Watch what you eat" is not comprehensive nutrition guidance.

All pregnant women require a similar level of protein and nutrients such as calcium and iron. In *The Pregnancy Diet,* women will learn how to meet their need for these essential nutrients, using a menu based on the National Research Council's nutrient and energy recommendations for pregnant women. However, these general guidelines will not apply to all women at all times. Calorie needs can vary from woman to woman for obvious reasons. The tall, active woman will require more energy than the short, sedentary woman, and the mother carrying twins needs more to eat than the mother carrying one baby. With the help of her doctor and *The Pregnancy Diet,* a woman can develop a weight-gain target and an eating plan that will meet her specific needs. The eating plan I recommend for pregnant women is based on six food groups, using delicious whole foods. There is even room for your favorite dietary indulgences to make it officially okay for you and baby to have a treat once in a while!

Pregnancy provides a wonderful opportunity to take care of yourself. At no other time are you likely to see a physician (or other health-care provider) quite so often. You are expected to want and need good food. Colleagues will not admonish you for eating an afternoon snack and spouses are more likely to indulge quirky cravings if they develop. It is during this time (and the postpartum period as well) that many family habits take shape, so use this opportunity to develop routines that will support everyone's good health. Make it a priority to eat fresh, wholesome food, to relax when you need to, and to move your body in some form of physical activity every day. Don't make the mistake of thinking you're being selfish for taking extra care of yourself; your child will most certainly reap the many benefits from your good health.

In my career as a nutritionist I have talked to many women about food, weight, and pregnancy. Pregnancy is not the time to diet, and this book is not intended to be used as a means for weight control. Rather it is a guide for women who want to make smart, informed choices about what they eat when they are pregnant and after. This book can be used by all pregnant women, but it will be particularly helpful and reassuring to those who are concerned about gaining too much or too little weight while pregnant.

1

Heavy Issues

Many people believe that pregnancy contributes to obesity. However, research shows that women who gain as recommended while they are pregnant have no greater reason to fear a permanent battle with obesity than nonpregnant women of the same age. Instead, pregnant women should take comfort in knowing that by gaining that recommended 25 to 35 pounds they have made an important contribution to the health of their baby.

HOW MUCH WEIGHT

The current weight gain recommendations for women of normal weight during pregnancy are at a higher level than they have been in the past 20 to 30 years. In the 1960s, the typical expectant mother was told to limit her weight gain to 15 to 20 pounds. She was even encouraged to use appetite suppressants and low-calorie diets to limit her weight gain, thereby preventing weight-related health problems and making her delivery easier. In the 1970s, researchers saw a connection between low weight gain and the birth of pre-term, low-birth-weight babies. As a result, the 1970s mom was told to gain 20 to 25 pounds. In the 1980s researchers saw a 20 percent reduction in low-birth-weight babies among white mothers and a 7 percent reduction among black mothers who gained eight to ten pounds more than their 1970s counterparts. As a result, weight-gain recommendations were increased even further. Today, the Institute of Medicine (IOM) offers a general weight-gain recommendation during pregnancy of 25 to 35 pounds, plus three different weight-gain guidelines based on a woman's weight for height before conception.

Weight-gain ranges are based on prepregnancy *body mass index* (BMI). BMI is defined as *body weight divided by height squared,* and it is considered a better indicator of nutritional status than weight alone. Use your prepregnancy weight to calculate your BMI with the help of the chart on page 3. Once you determine your prepregnancy BMI, select the interpretation that describes you: underweight, normal, overweight, or obese. A 5′8″ woman weighing 140 pounds at conception has a "normal" BMI of 21.5. A 5′8″ woman weighing 120 pounds, with a BMI of less than 19 is described as "underweight." Once your BMI is determined, select the recommended weight gain that matches your description.

Determining Body Mass Index from Height and Weight

Weight (lbs.) by BMI

Ht (ft'in)	19	20	21	22	23	24	25	26	27	28	29	30	35	40
4'10	91	96	100	105	110	115	119	124	129	134	138	143	167	191
4'11	94	99	104	109	114	119	124	128	133	138	143	148	173	198
5'0	97	102	107	112	118	123	128	133	138	143	148	153	179	204
5'1	100	106	111	116	122	127	132	137	143	148	153	158	185	211
5'2	104	109	115	120	126	131	136	142	147	153	158	164	191	218
5'3	107	113	118	124	130	135	141	146	152	158	163	169	197	225
5'4	110	116	122	128	134	140	145	151	157	163	169	174	204	232
5'5	114	120	126	132	138	144	150	156	162	168	174	180	210	240
5'6	118	124	130	136	142	148	155	161	167	173	179	186	216	247
5'7	121	127	134	140	146	153	159	166	172	178	185	191	223	255
5'8	125	131	138	144	151	158	164	171	177	184	190	197	230	262
5'9	128	135	142	149	155	162	169	176	182	189	196	203	236	270
5'10	132	139	146	153	160	167	174	181	193	200	208	215	250	286
5'11	136	143	150	157	165	172	179	186	193	200	208	215	250	286
6'0	140	147	154	162	169	177	184	191	199	206	213	221	258	294
6'1	144	151	159	166	174	182	189	197	204	212	219	227	265	302
6'2	148	155	163	171	179	186	194	202	210	218	225	233	272	311
6'3	152	160	168	176	184	192	200	208	216	224	232	240	279	319
6'4	156	164	172	180	189	197	205	213	221	230	238	246	287	328

Source: G. A. Bray, D. S. Gray. "Obesity, Part I, Pathogenesis." *Western Journal of Medicine* 149:429–441, 1988. Reproduced with permission.

To use this table, find your height in the left column, then move across that row to your weight. The number at the top of that column is your body mass index.

Recommended Weight Gain Based on BMI

These are general guidelines developed by the IOM. Your health-care team may adjust these recommendations based on your medical history and past pregnancy experience.

BMI	Recommended Total Weight Gain
Underweight (BMI<19.8)	28–40 pounds
Normal weight (BMI 19.8–26.0)	25–35 pounds
Overweight (BMI 26–29)	15–25 pounds
Obese (BMI>29)	15+ pounds

HOW FAST SHOULD I GAIN?

Your doctor will weigh you at every visit. Some women hate these weight checks and feel they are the doctor's way of checking up on them to see whether they have been "good" or "bad." The truth is that your doctor *is* checking up on you, but only to look for signs of good or bad health. Weight can be a very effective tool when evaluating the progress of a pregnancy.

A gradual, steady weight gain is ideal. In the first 13 weeks most obstetricians like to see a weight gain of two to five pounds, followed by a steady increase of approximately one pound per week until delivery. A gradual gain in weight suggests that both lean and fat tissue are being added, whereas an erratic and sudden increase can indicate a dangerous problem, such as the retention of fluid that is one of the symptoms of preeclampsia (see page 149).

Though the ideal might be a nice, steady, even weight gain, in reality most women will not gain weight in such a uniform manner. The *British Journal of Obstetrics and Gynecology* published a 1991 study that took a retrospective look at how mothers with a normal pregnancy outcome gain weight, and found that there was a wide variation in weight gain over the course of pregnancy. The slowest weight gain occurred before 16 weeks, after 35 weeks, and right before the eighth month between week 28 and week 32. The differences in average weekly weight gain among the mothers studied were related to number of pregnancies, BMI, smoking habits, and history of high blood pressure.

Many things can make it difficult to interpret weight gain. If the date of conception is uncertain, it is difficult to assess weight-gain patterns. In some cases, an unexpected weight gain can be related to how much food or liquid was consumed before a weight check. Whether a mother has a full or empty bladder or has had a bowel movement will affect the recorded weight. Even clothing and time of day affect weight measurements. The point is, a jump in weight does not always mean you ate too much or that something is wrong. In some cases it is a fluke in the weighing technique. As always, talk to your health-care provider and focus on the trend in weight gain, not just one reading.

To help practitioners and women make sense of what is considered a healthy weight-gain trend, the IOM has suggested the recommended weight-gain patterns listed on page 6. With the help of your doctor, use these to establish a weight-gain goal that is right for you.

Recommended Weight Gain Patterns

BMI	First Trimester Total	Weekly Weight Gain, Weeks 14–40
Normal weight	3.5 pounds	slightly less than 1 pound/week
Underweight	5 pounds	slightly more than 1 pound/week
Overweight	2 pounds	approximately ⅔ pound/week

Adolescent women need to aim for the high end of the recommended weight ranges, and women under 5′2″ should attempt to keep to the lower end. Women who are carrying twins may be advised to gain 35 to 45 pounds. The IOM suggests that women of normal weight who gain less that two pounds per month should investigate the reasons for slow weight gain with their doctor. And women who do not gain at least ten pounds by midpregnancy need to receive nutrition counselling. Gains of over six and a half pounds per month may need to be monitored, but food intake should not automatically be reduced. Weight gain continues to be important until the end of pregnancy. For instance, a low weight gain in normal-weight women in the last three months of pregnancy may be a cause of early delivery.

What Is All That Weight Made Of?

The weight you gain is not all baby, nor all fat. Just look where it goes:

	Weight (lbs.)
Fetus	7.5–8.5
Fat and protein stores	7.5
Blood	4.0
Tissue fluids	2.7
Uterus	2.0
Amniotic fluid	1.8
Placenta and umbilical cord	1.5
Breasts	1.0
Total	28–29

Is gaining above the recommended weight-gain levels even better for baby? The answer is, probably not. In a study of over 53,000 infants it was found that low birth weight decreased with increasing weight gain in average-weight women, but there was no further reduction in low birth weight when weight gains were higher than 30 to 40 pounds. Women with high weight gains are at increased risk for high-birth-weight babies, which can make delivery difficult. If you have a BMI higher than 29 you may be advised by your doctor to limit your weight gain to 15 to 25 pounds. (Some physicians may recommend an even lower weight gain based on a woman's medical history.) A lower weight gain may reduce an overweight woman's risk for a high-birth-weight infant.

AFTER DELIVERY

No one can predict exactly how any individual woman will gain or lose weight but a review of the research can give mothers some reassuring news. In 1993, Sally Ann Lederman, Ph.D., then of Columbia University's School of Public Health, reviewed the pregnancy-related research to determine whether one's weight increases permanently as a result of pregnancy. The studies showed that the average woman generally retains less than three pounds of added weight (from before pregnancy to one year after delivery). A small number of women may retain a lot of their pregnancy weight, but this is more likely due to having been overweight at conception and to lifestyle changes rather than to pregnancy itself. The woman who begins her pregnancy overweight may be at greater risk for being heavier after delivery.

A study of 1,423 Swedish mothers who averaged the recommended 30-pound gain during pregnancy found that the average weight gain was only three pounds one year after delivery. In another study the weight-gain patterns of 795 American women who gained approximately 28 pounds during pregnancy were examined. It was found that they averaged only three pounds above their initial weight at their six-month postpartum visit. This research suggests that for an average-weight woman, weight retention related to pregnancy is about three pounds, six months to one year after delivery. It is important to note that there are big differences among the women in these studies. In the Swedish study, for example, 2 percent of the mothers gained 20 pounds from before pregnancy to one year after delivery. The women gaining the most weight tended to be overweight to begin with.

Being Overweight Before Pregnancy

Women who are overweight before pregnancy can benefit by setting weight-gain goals for their pregnancy with their doctor. In a study that looked back on the weight gains of 128 severely obese women, more than 70 percent of these mothers had retained over 20 pounds one year after delivery. This suggests that for the very overweight woman, pregnancy can contribute significantly to weight. In another study at the University of Utah the weight histories of 96 very obese mothers were compared to 115 non-obese women. It was observed that the obese mothers had gained *100 pounds* by age 46 and the control group 31 pounds. The obese women retained more weight after their first pregnancy than the control group, and the obese women lost less weight after delivery and had greater gains between pregnancies than did the control group. (It may be that women who end up obese increase weight gradually over 20 years and some of that time pregnancy is happening.)

Women who gain excessive weight during pregnancy may increase their chance of induced labor and risk for an emergency cesarean section. Research suggests that obese women are more likely to have large babies no matter what their weight gain.

If you are overweight before pregnancy you may be at greater risk for retaining weight postpartum. With the help of your medical team, develop a weight-gain goal while pregnant and a weight-loss plan following delivery. The woman who begins her pregnancy overweight is at the greatest risk for being even heavier after delivery and will benefit most by considering her food selections very carefully.

Aging

For most women it is not pregnancy that is the cause of weight gain, but rather the fact they are getting older. In a study of over 41,184 postmenopausal women, even the women who had no children gained a significant amount of weight between ages 18 and 50. In this study, the difference in weight between women who had no children and those who had one to four children was small. In a large Finnish study that compared the weight of women with and without children, women who were over 35 and had no children weighed more than younger women who had had several children. It is not childbirth but aging that appears to explain the creeping weight many women experience.

Age has a bigger effect on weight than having children does, but women who have more than three children do tend to be heavier than women of the same age who have fewer children. This weight difference may not be due to pregnancy alone but may be the result of women having some of their children when they are older, when weight retention seems more common. Studies show that women over age 35 are more likely to retain greater weight after pregnancy than younger mothers.

The study on postmenopausal women suggests that as we age we can expect to gain about three-quarters of a pound per year. That's almost four pounds every five years, or 16 pounds in 20 years. This weight gain occurs independently of whether a woman has children or not.

In a 1994 report, Dr. D. F. Williamson looked at the weight history of 2,547 women age 25 to 45 who participated in the first National Health and Nutrition Examination Survey. These women were weighed in the early 1970s, then again ten years later. In that ten-year period, the women who had not had children had gained 3.52 pounds, the women who had had up to two children had gained 3.74 pounds, and the mother with three children had gained 4.84 pounds. There is a difference in weight gain, but it is very modest and means women do not need to fear a life of obesity just because they decide to become mothers.

Higher Weight-gain Guidelines

The weight-gain recommendations are now set higher for most women than they were before and some women may wonder if this increases the chance of permanent weight gain. The Institute of Medicine's weight-gain guidelines of 25 to 35 pounds are a good five to ten pounds above the 1970 guidelines of 20 to 25 pounds. The additional weight gain increases the birth weight of babies at delivery, which decreases infant mortality but may also create a degree of apprehension among women who fear permanent weight gain by meeting these higher recommendations. In 1993, Kenneth Keppel, Ph.D., of the National Center for Health Statistics, examined the actual weight retention among women who reached these higher guidelines. Women were interviewed 10 to 18 months after delivery. At that time, the median weight for white women who gained as recommended was 1.6 pounds higher than their weight before pregnancy, for black women it was 7.2 pounds. Thus, white women who gain the recommended amount of weight do not need to fear retaining a substantial amount of weight; however black women are at greater risk for being heavier after delivery, perhaps because they are not getting accurate information about weight gain recommendations during pregnancy and they may need advice on how to lose weight following delivery.

CHANGING LIFESTYLES

Anyone who has a baby will experience lifestyle changes she never imagined. The mother who goes from full-time office worker to full-time, stay-at-home mom may find weight an issue for the first time. This is less the result of pregnancy, and more due to the access she now has to food and the reduced opportunity to exercise.

A 1992 study by Dr. C. W. Schauberger that examined the factors that influence postpartum weight loss found that women who delayed returning to work were likely to gain more weight than women who returned to work sooner. Women who returned to work two weeks after delivery were only one pound above their weight before pregnancy when they were examined six months after delivery. Women who did not return to paid work were almost five pounds heavier at six months postpartum.

This is important because it is estimated that more than half of new mothers do not work outside the home in the first year of their baby's life. Women who stay at home have more frequent contact with food and are often responsible for preparing meals for the family. It is important to identify the lifestyle changes pregnancy creates and the effect they can have on weight.

Lifestyle can be modified to meet healthful eating goals. For example, keep the cupboards stocked with healthful snacks, not high-calorie snack foods like chips and cookies. Start an exercise routine that works for you; find something you like and do it every day. Keep food out of sight and eat only when hungry or in designated areas such as the kitchen table—not in front of the TV.

Another factor that affects postpartum weight is smoking. Fortunately, about 15 percent of pregnant women quit smoking on their own and another 40 percent will do so if encouraged by their family and physician. Quitting the habit improves the growth of the baby inside the mother, but women who quit smoking while pregnant may have a higher, but not necessarily excessive, weight gain. If you have quit smoking, congratulate yourself! Not only will it be good for your health, it will be good for the baby, both before birth and later, growing up in a smoke-free environment. If you have quit, you may have to be extra attentive to your eating and exercise habits after the baby is born to adapt to your new lifestyle.

BREAST-FEEDING

Breast-feeding has been touted as an effective method for controlling weight postpartum. Breast-feeding is the ideal way for most women to feed their baby, but its effect on weight loss is not as great as was once thought. Dr. Lederman's review concluded that at six months postpartum, weight loss was greater for breast-feeding mothers, but at 12 months postpartum, there was no significant difference in weight between breast-feeding mothers and mothers who bottlefed their baby. However, the studies have shown that mothers who breast-feed can lose weight even if they are not dieting, while those who choose to bottlefeed have to reduce what they eat if they want to take off extra pounds.

Breast-feeding women require more calories while nursing, about 500 extra calories per day. This means they can eat more food because they also need more in order to meet the demands of making breast milk. Breast-feeding deserves to be promoted for the indisputable health benefits it can provide to your child, but it does not guarantee that you will lose weight. You may still need to match what you eat to fit your new life pattern. Read more about breast-feeding, diet, and exercise in Chapter 7.

EATING DISORDERS AND PREGNANCY

Though eating disorders and pregnancy have not been well researched, there is enough information to offer comfort and guidance on this issue. It is estimated that 1 percent of general practice patients are bulimic (a binge-purge pattern) and up to 2 percent of young women could be affected by anorexia nervosa (a disorder characterized by starvation, distorted body image, and extreme fear of obesity). Women who suffer from anorexia nervosa are less likely to become pregnant than women with bulimia, in part because anorexia nervosa results in a lower fertility rate, caused by very low body weight, and in part because women with this condition are usually less sexually active.

Eating disorders during pregnancy hold the potential for disaster. Women with eating disorders are often underweight at conception, increasing the risk of delivering a low-birth-weight infant. Obstetricians have reported increased rates of difficult labor among these women requiring medical intervention. A child born to a mother with an uncontrolled eating disorder may be at greater risk for early or breech delivery, cleft palate, and delayed development.

The news about eating disorders is not all gloomy, however. In a review of the clinical significance of eating disorders during pregnancy, Thomas A. Fahy has found that bulimic women show a temporary improvement in their binging and purging behavior during the late stages of pregnancy. In a study of 20 untreated women, 75 percent had stopped this behavior by the third trimester. However, symptoms did return after delivery and, in half the cases, eating habits were more disturbed. It is important to emphasize that these women were not in treatment for their disorders. In one case a bulimic woman had recurrent miscarriages between the third and fifth month. When the disorder was in remission, she was able to deliver two full-term infants. In another eating-disorder observation, eight women, who had been afflicted with anorexia nervosa but gained an adequate amount of weight while pregnant, delivered healthy babies of normal weight. Seven of these women were in psychiatric treatment before or during pregnancy.

For any woman who is afflicted with an eating disorder, treatment and remission are important to a healthy pregnancy. The woman with an eating disorder who gains adequate weight will go a long way toward reducing her risk of pregnancy complications and improving the health of her child.

EATING DISORDERS AND PARENTING

An active disorder has the potential to be damaging while a woman is pregnant but the impact on the child does not stop there. Mothers who fear food and are intensely preoccupied with their body will experience conflicts with their own maternal responsibilities to feed and nurture appropriately. In a Danish study 17 percent of the babies born to women with anorexia nervosa showed failure to thrive in the first year. For bulimic mothers, the energy devoted to the rituals of planning and executing binges may take away from the time they spend parenting. In a study of the children of five bulimic women, the mothers had undue concern about weight, and the children were not well nourished.

In a review of this issue, Debra Franko, Ph.D., director of the Eating Disorder Program at the Harvard-affiliated Beth

Israel Hospital states that shame, secrecy, and denial prevent women from sharing their problem with their doctors. In an ideal world, women would be asked about eating disorders during their prenatal exams and referred to a psychiatrist or an eating disorder clinic when a problem is identified. Research shows that women with eating disorders in remission or in treatment significantly reduce their complications.

Women who are aware of their eating disorders should also become aware of the weight gain recommended for their BMI. If you are underweight before conception, make a special effort to meet the recommended goals. Reread the beginning of this chapter to understand that weight gained during pregnancy is not permanent in the majority of women. Join a pregnancy support group or a pregnancy exercise class. These can be lots of fun and will give you an opportunity to discuss your fears and validate the feelings that come with pregnancy. Seek out a therapist who is trained in eating disorders. Having someone to share your feelings with can be helpful.

If you have an eating disorder it is just as important to take care of yourself after the baby is born. Join a parenting class. Get a few good books on feeding your baby and on the normal development of children. (There are some recommended titles in the back of this book.) In a culture that is obsessed with thinness some parents control food so much that they actually deprive their children of the food they need.

PUTTING THE WEIGHT ISSUE TOGETHER

Research shows that women who gain an average amount of weight while pregnant can expect to retain about two pounds above and beyond their expected weight increase with age. Women who gain significantly above their recommended levels are likely to retain more postpartum. Women who are the thinnest before conception should gain the most; underweight women should gain 28 to 40 pounds during their pregnancy. Proper weight gain is of most concern to thin women who are restricting their food intake. Women who do not eat enough cannot achieve nutrient balance. Early weight is important for the growth of the baby later and normalized maternal weight will optimize that growth, which is important to prevent restricted brain and organ development, and to optimize health.

Pregnancy itself does not lead to obesity except in a small percentage of women. Reaching the desired weight gain appropriate for your size is important. While pregnant, staying in the weight range developed between you and your doctor may be helpful in preventing a postpartum weight problem. You cannot predict or control how your body gains weight while you are pregnant, and every pregnancy (even each of yours) will be different—just ask your doctor. Your responsibility is to eat well and eat the foods you need for good health. When you eat well, exercise appropriately, and rest as needed, your body will do all the work of building your baby.

The most common nutritional concern of women during pregnancy is excessive weight gain. However with realistic weight goals and a healthful eating plan, these fears about excessive weight gain do not need to become reality.

2

Nutrition Basics

The wonderful opportunity of pregnancy, besides having a baby, is that you are expected to take extra care of yourself, and even allowed to indulge in some self-pampering. It is a time when you can tell your family and friends that you need to rest, walk, relax, or even nap and they are apt to accommodate you or at least understand. Women are likely to focus on nutrition now more than at any other time in their lives. This newfound respect for nutrition is certainly good news for your growing baby, but, just as importantly, it is good news for you. This is especially true if you have been, like so many women, not so thoughtful about what you ate until you became pregnant.

It is estimated that, at any given time, 40 percent of American women have been on a weight-reducing diet in the past five to six months. These diets are usually below 1,500 calories and low in essential nutrients. In addition, at least one government survey has found that 50 to 60 percent of women do not eat enough of the right foods to meet the Recommended Dietary Allowances (RDAs) for all nutrients. This means that about half of the women reading this book really do need to improve their eating habits.

The woman who begins her pregnancy poorly nourished can increase her chances of iron deficiency, fatigue, and a low-birth-weight baby. At least one study found that good nutrition during pregnancy can protect against high blood pressure in children tested at age 11. This suggests that your diet can have a far-reaching role in your child's health.

The good news is that a woman's body, as soon as she is pregnant, will become more efficient and effective at retaining nutrients. In fact, most of the changes you will experience while pregnant occur to improve the efficiency of nutrient absorption. For example, in the third month of pregnancy, metabolic and circulation rates increase so the nutrients you eat can be easily passed to your baby. Blood volume will increase by half to accommodate the nutrients and waste products that travel from mother to fetus and back again. The increased need for sleep that almost all mothers experience, sometimes as the first sign of pregnancy, is believed to be a way your body conserves energy.

Much of the weight you gain will be from the development of the amniotic sac and the growth of the uterus and its supporting muscles. Breasts will change and grow in preparation for lactation. To provide for the energy needed at birth and through the first months postpartum, the pregnant woman will store approximately 7.5 pounds of needed fat, an amount theoretically capable of yielding over 26,000 calories. Look to page 7 for a breakdown of where weight is distributed during pregnancy.

Use your doctor appointments to monitor and evaluate how well you are meeting eating and exercising goals. Use the medical team for reassurance and weight checks. Consider keeping a monthly notebook. A pregnancy journal is a great place to write questions for the doctor and personal health goals, plus it makes a wonderful keepsake.

HEALTHY BEGINNINGS

Even if weight is your biggest food worry, concerns about supplements, morning sickness, constipation, and heartburn are likely to come up as well. In most cases the eating recommendations for a healthy pregnancy will keep weight gain at an appropriate level and help ease the food-associated problems that can accompany pregnancy. Good nutrition, a healthy lifestyle, and a gradual, steady weight gain are your first important tasks as a mother. These are not hard to accomplish if you follow these simple guidelines.

◎ Get early and regular prenatal care. Expect to make 10 to 14 doctor visits during each pregnancy.

◎ Do not consume alcohol.

◎ Do not smoke.

◎ Before taking any medication while pregnant, consult your physician (this includes nonprescription pills as well).

◎ Establish a weight-gain goal with your health-care provider and meet it. Adequate weight gain is one of the most effective ways to insure a healthy pregnancy. Read more about this on page 67.

◎ Continue (or establish) an appropriate exercise routine.

◎ Eat a variety of food:

　　3 to 5 servings of fruit or juice each day.

　　2 to 4 servings of vegetables daily.

　　7 to 11 servings of bread/starch daily.

　　2 to 3 servings of protein-rich foods.

　　3 to 4 servings of calcium-rich foods.

- Eat small moderate meals to promote comfort and nutrition.

- For iron, include some meat, poultry, or fish daily (and add a food rich in vitamin C, which helps your body absorb iron).

- Consume sweets, sugars, and soft drinks in moderation.

- Consume salt and salty foods in moderation, but don't *restrict* salt—your need for salt increases while you are pregnant.

- Drink coffee or other caffeinated beverages in moderation, two to three servings or less per day.

- Ask your doctor about the need for vitamin/mineral supplements.

If you follow the above guidelines you will be doing exactly what you and your baby need to create a healthy pregnancy.

SPECIAL EATING PROBLEMS

Just when nutrition becomes so important it seems as though pregnancy simultaneously creates eating problems such as nausea, vomiting, constipation, and heartburn. All these are normal pregnancy experiences that cannot be avoided entirely, but understanding why they occur and how food affects them may help you worry less and develop healthy habits.

Morning Sickness

Morning sickness occurs between the fifth and sixteenth week of pregnancy, and it affects at least half of all pregnancies, especially first-time mothers. The symptoms of nausea and vomiting known as morning sickness are often a woman's first confirming sign of pregnancy. But, be advised that these symptoms are not necessarily confined to the morning. The precise cause of morning sickness remains unknown but one suspected trigger is the hormone called *human chorionic gonadotropin* (HCG), which is produced by the placenta and governs changes in estrogen and progesterone production during the first trimester of pregnancy.

The good news about morning sickness is that it is normal and a good sign. A study by the National Institute of Child Health and Human Development and the National Institute of Allergy and Infectious Disease found that women who vomit during their pregnancy are less likely to miscarry or deliver prematurely than women who don't. Nevertheless it is still an unpleasant experience and one you will want to control if possible.

In a small percentage of women (3.5 per 1,000 pregnancies) the nausea and vomiting can become so severe and protracted that it progresses to a condition called *hyperemesis* and requires medical treatment. This condition can be successfully treated, but regular checkups will ensure that a case of severe morning sickness is dealt with before it progresses that far.

In the 1940s, studies suggested that vitamin B_6 could help relieve morning sickness, but a 1979 review of the issue by the American Medical Council on Drugs stated that there was no evidence vitamin B_6 could effectively treat nausea and this view was substantiated again in a 1986 report. Only under the care of a physician should vitamin B_6, also known as pyridoxine, be taken during pregnancy.

For most women there will be no need for medical treatment of morning sickness. Women should take reassurance in the fact that time is on their side, and symptoms will almost always abate on their own, usually by the end of the first trimester.

The Benefits of Ginger for Morning Sickness

Ginger is credited with treating nausea. Try it in the form of ginger ale, ginger tea, or ginger tablets available at the health-food store. Do not take more than four 250-mg. doses per day, and if you use ginger tablets for more than four days in a row to control nausea, make sure that your doctor is alerted.

Follow these tips to relieve morning sickness:

- ◎ Eat small, frequent meals.
- ◎ Carbohydrate foods such as rice, plain potatoes, or sliced bread may be better tolerated than other foods.
- ◎ Try snacking on saltine crackers, pretzels, or dry toast before getting out of bed.
- ◎ Try drinking liquids between meals, not with meals.
- ◎ Gelatin desserts such as flavored Jell-O may be well tolerated. Gelatin is a good source of fluids.
- ◎ Some women may find relief drinking sugared, decaffeinated, or herbal teas and nondiet ginger ale.
- ◎ Avoid citrus drinks first thing in the morning.
- ◎ Avoid strong smells like burned toast, brewed coffee, cigarette smoke, and cooking smells.
- ◎ Avoid extreme food temperatures: no frozen or steaming-hot food items.

◉ Avoid foods that are fried or are rich in added fats like mayonnaise or butter.

◉ Make the time to practice deep breathing as a form of relaxation therapy before meals.

◉ Some women find that prenatal supplements aggravate morning sickness. Discuss their discontinuance with your doctor.

◉ In a 1992 study acupressure helped 60 percent of pregnant women who had nausea and vomiting. Women can find acupressure wrist bands at boating stores and travel clubs such as an AAA autoclub.

◉ Miriam Erick, author of *No More Morning Sickness*, recommends that if none of these food approaches work, eat whatever you can keep down—that might even include a traditional no-no like potato chips.

Cravings

A 1985 study found that 76 percent of the pregnant women surveyed reported a craving for at least one food item and that 85 percent reported an aversion to at least one food item. The cause and effect of food cravings is not known, but its overall effect on nutrition is probably not significant. One exception is the food craving known as *pica*, which can indicate a serious nutrition problem. Pica is a severe form of iron deficiency that exerts unusual cravings for nonfood items such as ice, dirt, or even detergent. If you find yourself with this sort of craving, call it to the attention of your doctor. A blood test will indicate if there is a nutritional problem, which in most cases is very easy to correct. In general it is safe to indulge your food cravings as long as you are eating the core foods you need for good nutrition and are not going overboard on the total amount of foods you eat.

Constipation

If you have seen a medical illustration of a full-term baby in its mother's womb you will understand why mothers experience digestive problems, including constipation. In the last weeks of your pregnancy the baby will be nestled snug in the uterus, which has grown along with the baby. At five months the baby is about eight inches long and only half a pound, and at seven months she is 12 inches long and now weighs two or three pounds. As the baby grows to full size, the entire digestive tract is compressed to make way for this temporary visitor. As the baby pushes on the stomach, heartburn can result, and as the intestines get crowded, constipation and flatulence occur. Not only does the enlarged uterus make elimination difficult, but the placental hormones relax gastrointestinal muscles, further adding to the potential problem of constipation. Constipation is a normal experience of pregnancy but there are ways to make things better:

◉ Drink enough fluids. Fill a one-quart jug of water each morning and make a serious effort to finish it that same day.

◉ Eat plenty of fiber: at least three whole-grain foods per day (this includes whole-grain cereal, brown rice, whole-wheat bread) plus the recommended number of fruits and vegetables, at least equaling five or more each day.

◉ Take time to go to the bathroom. When you have the urge to go, don't put it off.

◉ Do not take laxatives unless they are prescribed by your doctor.

✆ Iron supplements are a frequent cause of constipation. If you are not anemic you may be able to meet your iron needs through dietary sources of iron, which do not cause constipation. Discuss the elimination of the iron supplement with your doctor.

Heartburn

Heartburn becomes a problem later in pregnancy as the baby grows. Your stomach and your enlarging baby will both share the same crowded area. The enlarged uterus puts pressure on the stomach, causing some of the stomach contents to move up into the esophagus, the tube that connects the mouth and stomach. This causes a "burning" sensation known as heartburn. The problem has no connection to the heart except by proximity (and it does not mean the baby's hair is rubbing against the heart or stomach either!). Here are some tips for heartburn:

✆ Eat small frequent meals. Try a schedule of three small meals and three small snacks.

✆ Drink liquids before or after meals instead of with meals. This will help to keep the contents in the stomach smaller, which may help to lessen the symptoms.

✆ Wear loose-fitting clothes.

✆ Avoid high-fat foods such as fried items or those with rich sauces, butter, or mayonnaise.

✆ Do not lie down right after meals.

Hemorrhoids

Hemorrhoids are enlarged veins in the anus that protrude through the anal sphincter. They usually occur in the later

part of pregnancy. Pregnant women get hemorrhoids because of the increased weight of the baby and the down-
ward pressure it causes on the lower intestine. Hemorrhoids can be painful and cause burning and itching. If they
rupture, they can cause bleeding, which is often more
alarming than serious. Here are a few tips to prevent or
treat hemorrhoids:

⑨ Prevent constipation by following the advice about fluids
  and fiber recommended earlier.

⑨ Every afternoon, and more often if you need it, put your
  feet up and rest. This will take pressure off of your
  digestive tract.

PRENATAL VITAMINS

Because the nutritional demands are so great during pregnancy most women assume they need supplements. It may
surprise you to learn that neither the Food and Nutrition
Board nor the American College of Obstetricians and Gynecologists recommend the routine use of supplements during
pregnancy for women eating a balanced diet. The only
women who are actually advised to supplement their diet
when pregnant are women who do not normally eat properly, who are carrying more than one fetus, who are heavy
smokers, or who abuse drugs and alcohol. Women who have
previously delivered a low-birth-weight baby and have only a
short gap between pregnancies may be advised to take
supplements, too. Despite the lack of an across-the-board
recommendation, as many as 92 percent of pregnant women
take vitamin supplements during their pregnancy.

Supplements are not always harmless. In a 1988 report

on vitamins the American Academy of Pediatrics and American College of Obstetricians and Gynecologists wrote: "It is important to avoid excessive vitamin and mineral intakes (i.e., more than twice the recommended dietary allowances) during pregnancy because both fat-soluble and water-soluble vitamins may have toxic effects." The nutrients that can potentially become toxic include iron, zinc, selenium, and vitamins A, B_6, C, and D. These nutrients are discussed below, along with vitamin B_{12}, folate, and calcium, which are nutrients that are often recommended during pregnancy. Always inform your doctor of all vitamin and mineral pills you take.

Nutrient-Nutrient Interactions

Aside from their potential toxicity when taken in large amounts, nutrients also need to be taken carefully in case they interfere with each other. Using the chart below, you can see that taking one nutrient can impact on the effect of another, compromising their benefits. What this means is that a woman taking extra iron may actually cause a decrease in the zinc she absorbs, or a woman who takes extra calcium may cause a reduction in iron absorption.

Iron can inhibit zinc absorption

Zinc can inhibit copper absorption

Calcium can interfere with iron

Protein increases urinary calcium losses

Protein increases vitamin B_6 requirements

Vitamin A Supplements

Vitamin A is toxic in large doses. Vitamin A, taken in the range of 25,000 international units (IU) or more daily, particularly in the first thirteen weeks, is associated with central nervous system abnormalities, altered growth, and a higher incidence of spontaneous abortion. Medication prescribed to treat acne may contain a derivative of vitamin A. These medications should be avoided by pregnant women as well as women planning to become pregnant. Discuss all medications with your doctor. Furthermore, vitamin A deficiency is rare in the United States, and studies indicate that U.S. women have an adequate store of vitamin A in their livers. Given that there is a risk for toxicity and little risk of vitamin A deficiency, routine supplementation with vitamin A is not recommended during pregnancy.

Vitamin B_6 Supplements

Adolescents, women carrying more than one baby, and women who abuse drugs and alcohol are at risk for being poorly nourished. Vitamin B_6 is an important nutrient that is easily obtained through food, but if you have any of the above situations a multivitamin supplement containing 2 mg. of B_6 is recommended by the National Research Council.

Vitamin B_{12} Supplements

Because this vitamin is abundant in meat, fish, eggs, and milk, it is only a concern for women who have avoided these foods for many years. In most cases, if women have eaten some of these foods in the years preceding pregnancy, they have stored enough B_{12} in their liver to last them for many years. A healthy baby is estimated to carry about 50 mcg. of B_{12}, and an adult mother stores approximately 3,000 mcg., so the drain on the mother's stores, in theory, should be slight. There have been isolated cases of babies being born with a B_{12} deficiency because of a mother's long-term vegan diet. For this reason the Subcommittee on Dietary Intake and Nutrients Supplements during Pregnancy recommends a daily vitamin B_{12} supplement of 2.0 mcg. daily for complete vegetarian women.

Vitamin C Supplements

This nutrient is one of the most frequently supplemented vitamins, and the risk of toxicity is low relative to the number of people who take it. Nevertheless vitamin C in megadoses (more than 3 grams per day) has resulted in side effects that include diarrhea and nausea, and can interfere with test results for diabetes and hemoglobin levels. Vitamin C is actively transported from the placenta to the baby's blood supply. A mother taking huge doses of vitamin C could markedly increase blood levels of vitamin C, creating a potentially harmful deficiency condition for her baby when supplementation is stopped (i.e. at birth). Do not supplement with vitamin C at doses that far exceed the RDA.

Vitamin D Supplements

If you are a woman who does not drink vitamin D–fortified milk, a supplement of 5 to 10 mcg. of vitamin D should be discussed with your doctor. Vitamin D is also received when the skin is exposed to sunlight so the risk of vitamin D deficiency increases during winter, when exposure to ultra-violet light decreases.

Folate Supplements

Neural tube defects (NTD) including anencephaly, spina bifida, and encephalocele are the most common birth defects. The cause is mostly unknown. However, observational studies have suggested that folic acid may prevent a portion of neural tube defects. In 1991, the Medical Research Council Vitamin Study Group found that folic acid given prior to and during pregnancy resulted in a 71 percent reduction in NTDs in patients who had previously given birth to a child with a NTD. The American College of Obstetricians and Gynecologists recommends that women with a NTD in a previous pregnancy should be offered treatment with folic acid before conception and continue through the first trimester. It should be noted that folic acid does not prevent all cases of NTD. The U.S. Public Health Service has recommended daily supplementation with 0.4 mg. (400 mcg.) of folic acid for all women who are capable of becoming pregnant. The public health department hopes to reduce the number of first occurrences of neural tube defects.

It is important for mothers to know that folic acid is important in preventing NTD *prior to* and *in the first four weeks* of pregnancy. During pregnancy, routine supplementation with folate is not recommended, but daily intake of fruits, vegetables, and whole grains (all sources of folate) is. See page 43 for sources of folic acid.

Calcium Supplements

Pregnant women who eat only one small dairy food per day are likely to get as little as 600 mg. of calcium from their total menu, which is about half of what is needed. If you eat only one calcium-rich food a day, add more milk, yogurt, cheese, or green leafy vegetables. If you can't increase your food sources of calcium, ask your doctor about taking a daily calcium supplement. Take the calcium supplement at mealtimes for better absorption and make sure you get enough vitamin D, which helps calcium absorption. Vitamin D can come from fortified milk, fortified breakfast cereal, multivitamins, and sun exposure.

Iron Supplements

Some women may begin their pregnancy with low iron stores, putting them at risk for a deficiency as the pregnancy progresses. The need for iron cannot be met by most women through diet alone. For this reason, iron in the second and third trimester is usually advised in a daily dose of 30 mg. of elemental ferrous iron daily. Iron can be obtained separately or in a prenatal supplement and should be taken between meals or at bedtime with water. This regimen is meant to prevent iron deficiency anemia. For information about iron deficiency anemia, see page 141 in Chapter 5.

Magnesium Supplements

It is estimated that 5 to 30 percent of all pregnant women may experience pregnancy-induced leg cramps. A randomized controlled trial of 73 pregnant women found that supplemental magnesium (122 mg. once in the morning and twice in the evening) was effective in reducing the incidence of leg cramps. There remains a concern, as with all supplements, that there may be a synergistic effect between multivitamins, iron supplements, and magnesium, which has not yet been examined. If leg cramps are a problem, discuss the use of supplemental magnesium with your doctor and keep in mind that you already get an amount of magnesium from your prenatal supplement.

Zinc Supplements

There is no need for routine supplementation during pregnancy, but when supplemental iron is taken in doses greater than 30 mg. per day, a zinc supplement is often recommended. Zinc taken in doses of 50 mg. of elemental zinc per day interfere with copper absorption, and when administered as a supplement it is recommended that a copper supplement at 2 mg. per day be included as well to compensate for the poor absorption.

THE BOTTOM LINE ON SUPPLEMENTS

If you are a pregnant woman in good health who eats well and is gaining an appropriate amount of weight, there is probably no need for you to take a nutrient supplement, except for iron at the 30 mg. range. If you are unable or unwilling to eat a balanced diet, or you have health issues that put you at risk, the Food and Nutrition Board of the Institute of Medicine suggests that you take a prenatal supplement that includes the following nutrients in the suggested doses.

VITAMIN	AMOUNT
B_6	2 mg.
Folate	300 mcg.
C	50 mg.
D	5 mcg.

MINERALS	
Iron	30 mg.
Zinc	15 mg.
Copper	2 mg.
Calcium	250 mg.

If you want to take a supplement "just in case" (and most women seem to), you are not likely to cause the baby any harm as long as you do not take supplements in large doses. According to *Modern Nutrition in Health and Disease*, edited by Maurice E. Shils, M.D., there is no evidence that multivitamin-mineral supplements will do any harm at a rate that does not exceed 1½ times the RDA. However, supplements are no replacement for a diet that includes a variety of foods. Remember, supplements carry no fiber, carbohydrate, or protein, which are nutrients that you and your baby will have to get from food. Keep your doctor informed of any supplements you take while pregnant.

NUTRITION SPECIFICS

All nutrients are important during pregnancy, but there are certain nutrients that mothers-to-be will want to give special attention. Your need for calcium, iron, and protein increases during pregnancy, and studies show that the intake of nutrients such as magnesium, the B complex (particularly

B_6), vitamin D, vitamin E, folic acid, zinc, and magnesium may be low in the diets of many women. What follows is a basic primer on the essential nutrients you need during pregnancy, including how much you need of each nutrient and advice on how to get these nutrients from food. Use this section as a reference and resource when you want information and reassurance about your food choices.

What are the RDAs?

The Recommended Dietary Allowances (RDAs) are recommended levels of essential nutrients established by the National Research Council and the National Academy of Sciences. These recommendations actually exceed the needs of most healthy people, meaning that when consumed at levels slightly below 100 percent of the RDA, a nutrient deficiency will not occur. The National Research Council has developed specific nutrient recommendations for pregnant women and this can be a useful tool to identify the nutrients and the foods pregnant women should eat. Before the discussion of each nutrient, the RDA for adult nonpregnant women is given, followed by the recommended RDA during pregnancy.

Protein

RDA: Adult women 50 grams; pregnant women 60 grams

Protein is essential for building muscle, organs, and healthy skin, as well as for making antibodies and hormones. More than 25 percent of the protein you eat while pregnant will go directly to the placenta and uterus. During pregnancy your daily need for protein increases by 10 grams. The usual intake of protein by pregnant American women is 75 to 110 grams per day, an amount that exceeds the established RDA. Approximately half of that protein will go to your baby, and it is estimated that during pregnancy a healthy mother will have given close to 1,000 grams of protein to her baby.

In the United States, protein deficiencies are rare. Symptoms can include skin lesions, brittle hair, and a low serum albumin level, which is detectable in blood tests. A mother's risk of protein malnutrition can be increased if she does not take in sufficient calories. When the body does not get enough energy food (carbohydrates), it will use protein as a source of fuel. This takes protein away from the growth processes (muscles, skin, hair, baby . . .) that are its primary function. For this reason, women must eat adequate amounts of protein as part of a diet that provides enough food overall to meet calorie needs. Most women have no difficulty obtaining the protein they need from food.

Good protein sources: Beef, chicken, pork, lamb, fish, milk, cheese, dried peas, beans, and grains.

Recommendations to meet your protein needs:

⑨ Eat the recommended amount of foods from the protein-rich group: approximately two servings or a total of 7 ounces of meat, fish, or chicken. One ounce of meat carries 7 grams of protein. Fish, chicken, pork, lamb, and beef are equal in protein content. A half-cup portion of cooked beans carries approximately 7 grams of protein.

⑨ Moderately increase your intake of breads, cereals, and starches to at least seven servings per day. Each serving carries about 2 grams of protein.

⑨ Moderately increase your intake of calcium-rich dairy foods to a total of three servings daily. One cup of milk or yogurt carries 8 grams of protein.

⑨ Eat enough food to meet your calorie needs, so the protein in your diet can be used by you and your baby for growth not fuel. Refer to Chapter 3 for information about determining your calorie needs.

⑨ Healthy pregnant women do not require protein supplements.

Vitamin E

RDA: Adult women 8 mg.; pregnant women 10 mg.

Vitamin E is an *antioxidant*, which means it traps the harmful byproducts of metabolism known as free radicals. In this way it helps protect our muscles, cardiovascular system, and nerve membranes. It also helps the body utilize vitamin A.

The RDA for Vitamin E increases slightly during pregnancy. Nutrition surveys have found that pregnant women consume about 3 to 9 mg. per day, an amount that falls below the RDA. Though women might not be getting the full RDA, there are no reports of definable deficiencies. Women who are on very-low-fat diets that exclude vegetable fats rich in vitamin E may be at the greatest risk for low vitamin E intake.

Good vitamin E sources: The richest sources are vegetable oils, such as cottonseed, safflower, corn, and soybean. Margarine, shortening, wheat germ, whole grains, and nuts are also good sources. (Vitamin E can be lost in processing, storage, and food preparation, so try to choose fresh, whole-food sources whenever possible.)

Recommendations to meet your vitamin E needs:

☯ Make at least three of your servings from the bread/starch group: whole-grain choices such as whole-wheat bread, whole-grain cereal, brown rice, and so on.

☯ Use at least one serving of vegetable oil daily in a salad dressing or in cooking. One teaspoon of corn oil carries 1 mg. of vitamin E. One teaspoon of sunflower oil carries 2 mg. of vitamin E.

☯ One tablespoon of wheat germ carries 20 mg. of vitamin E. Sprinkle it on cereal or over vegetables several times each week.

☯ One tablespoon of peanut butter carries 3 mg. of vitamin E. Choose it as a sandwich filling a couple of times a week.

Vitamin C

RDA: Adult women 60 mg.; pregnant women 70 mg.

Vitamin C may give us a slight edge when recovering from a cold, but its effect on iron is what makes it valuable. Vitamin C enhances iron absorption, and iron is much needed during pregnancy (read about iron on page 48). Like vitamin E and vitamin A, vitamin C is an antioxidant and may help prevent chronic disease.

During pregnancy the RDA increases by 10 mg. Food surveys indicate that American women consume in the range of 77 to 84 mg. of vitamin C each day, which is adequate. Women who use cigarettes, drugs, and alcohol are likely to have low blood levels of vitamin C. Women who have been long-term users of birth control pills or who take aspirin regularly may also need more vitamin C. There is no specific increase for women bearing twins or triplets, but it is recognized that women expecting multiple births are likely to require more vitamin C.

Good vitamin C sources: Vegetables and fruits are very good sources, particularly green and red peppers, collard greens, broccoli, spinach, tomatoes, potatoes, strawberries, oranges, limes, grapefruit, lemons. Meat, fish, poultry, eggs, and dairy foods carry very small amounts of vitamin C, and grains such as bread and cereal carry none.

Recommendations to meet your vitamin C needs:

⊚ Start your morning with a good vitamin C source, such as 4 ounces of orange juice; 4 ounces tomato juice; half a cup of strawberries; half a grapefruit. Each of these carry about 50 mg. of vitamin C.

⊚ Eat a total of three servings of fruit daily.

⊚ Eat two or more servings of vegetables daily.

⊚ Avoid overcooking fruits and vegetables—this can destroy nutrients.

Thiamin

RDA: Adult women 1.1 mg.; pregnant women 1.4 mg.

Thiamin, a member of the B complex group of vitamins, is essential to the proper metabolism of carbohydrate and energy production. The need for thiamin increases during pregnancy, in part to assist with the extra calories that will be eaten. It also helps keep the appetite and nervous system in good health.

Food surveys indicate that adult American women consume an average of 1.05 mg. of this nutrient daily. Increasing servings from the bread/starch group to meet the energy needs of pregnancy will allow women to meet the RDA for thiamin.

Good thiamin sources: All enriched breads, cereals, and grain products. Unrefined cereals, whole grains, brewer's yeast, organ meats (liver, heart, kidney), lean pork, legumes, seeds, and nuts.

Recommendations to meet your thiamin needs:

⑨ Increase your servings from the bread/starch group to the recommended level, eating at least seven servings per day.

⑨ Select enriched fortified cereal, rice, and breads. Grains carry an abundant supply of all the B complex nutrients. Each slice of bread carries approximately 0.1 mg., one serving of enriched cereal yields 0.4 mg. and ½ cup of cooked enriched rice carries 0.2 mg of thiamin.

Riboflavin

RDA: Adult women 1.1 mg.; pregnant women 1.4 mg.

Like thiamin, riboflavin is part of the nutrient group known as the B complex. It keeps skin healthy, promotes good vision, and helps in the release of food energy. Food surveys indicate that women consume about 1.34 mg. of riboflavin per day.

Good riboflavin sources: Meat, poultry, fish, and especially dairy products, including milk, yogurt, and cheese. Grains are naturally low in riboflavin, but most are enriched with the B vitamins, turning them into a great source of this vitamin.

Recommendations to meet your riboflavin needs:

◎ Be sure to get the recommended intake of dairy foods— at least three servings per day.

◎ Increase your bread/starch servings to the recommended level of at least seven per day.

◎ Shop for grains, cereals, and breads that are enriched with riboflavin.

Niacin

RDA: Adult women 14 mg.; pregnant women 18 mg.

Niacin is the collective name for nicotinic acid, nicotinamide, and niacinamide. Niacin is present in all cells and is essential to metabolism. It releases energy from food and keeps the skin and digestive tract healthy. Our need for niacin is so essential that the body creates an alternative source by converting the amino acid tryptophan to niacin. Tryptophan is abundant in milk and meat.

Adults consume about 27 mg. of niacin daily from tryptophan and preformed niacin. Because of its importance, a woman's ability to convert tryptophan to niacin increases while she is pregnant.

Good niacin sources: Meat carries large amounts of preformed niacin and tryptophan. Milk and eggs carry little niacin but they are a rich source of tryptophan, which can become a source of niacin. The niacin that is naturally present in cereal and grain products may not be well absorbed and is lost when milled or refined. In reality most of the niacin we use comes from the fully absorbable form of niacin that is added to fortified grain products like cereal and bread.

Recommendations to meet your niacin needs:

◎ Eat the recommended servings from the bread/starch group, at least seven servings per day.

◎ Eat the recommended servings from the protein-rich group, at least two servings per day.

Vitamin B₆ (pyridoxine)

RDA: Adult women 1.3 mg.; pregnant women 1.9 mg.

Vitamin B_6 is needed for proper metabolism of protein, carbohydrate, and fat. Because of the increased need for protein during pregnancy the requirement for B_6 increases too. This is also needed for proper immune-system and hormone function.

Clinical signs of B_6 deficiency are rare, but nutrition surveys often find that average intakes are in the 1.16 mg. range, below the RDA. A lack of vitamin B_6 has been linked with gestational diabetes and depression, but the accuracy of the studies making this connection have been challenged. Since most pregnant women take a multivitamin-mineral preparation containing B_6 it becomes easy to meet the requirement. *Beware:* large doses of vitamin B_6 can be toxic.

Supplements that exceed 500 mg. per day have been linked to side effects that include serious neurological damage.

Good vitamin B_6 sources: Best sources include chicken, fish, kidney, liver, pork, eggs. Good sources include un-milled rice, soybeans, oats, whole-wheat products, peanuts, and walnuts. Dairy products and red meats are relatively poor sources of vitamin B_6.

Recommendations to meet your vitamin B_6 needs:

- Eat the recommended two servings from the protein-rich group daily.
- Eat two to three eggs per week.

Folic Acid

RDA: Adult women 400 mcg.; pregnant women 600 mcg.

Folic acid, also known as folate and folacin, is used by the body to build new red blood cells. During pregnancy, folic acid has been found to reduce the risk of birth defects. (Read more about folic acid supplements and birth defects on page 31.) Because of its beneficial effect on the developing fetus, folic acid may eventually be added to grain products much in the way the B vitamins and iron are now added to cereals and grains.

Good folic acid sources: Green leafy vegetables, beans, seeds, liver, eggs, and wheat germ.

Recommendations to meet your folic acid requirements:

- Eat one type of dark green vegetable every day. Half a cup of cooked spinach carries 100 mcg.; half a cup of cooked broccoli, 50 mcg.

◎ Eat two to three servings of fruit daily. One orange carries 50 mcg.; one banana approximately 20 mcg.

◎ Eat two to three eggs per week. One egg carries 24 mcg.

◎ Sprinkle wheat germ on your breakfast cereal. One ounce (¼ cup) carries 100 mcg. of folic acid.

◎ Be careful while cooking vegetables. Overcooking can destroy folic acid.

◎ Storage can destroy folic acid. Wrap fresh produce and keep it refrigerated until you are ready to use it.

Vitamin B$_{12}$

RDA: Adult women 2.4 mcg.; pregnant women 2.6 mcg.

Vitamin B$_{12}$ is essential to normal cell division and protein synthesis. It works with other nutrients to make blood healthy. Without B$_{12}$ blood anemias will occur. Fortunately B$_{12}$ deficiencies are rare, occurring only when vitamin B$_{12}$ cannot be properly absorbed or when a very restricted diet that excludes meat, egg, or milk products is consumed for many years. Vegetarian women will have no trouble getting adequate amounts of B$_{12}$ if they consume either eggs, milk, or cheese, or fortified grains such as breakfast cereal.

Good vitamin B$_{12}$ sources: Meat, fish, eggs, milk and enriched grain products. Beans and nuts do not carry vitamin B$_{12}$.

Recommendations to meet your vitamin B$_{12}$ needs:

◎ Eat a daily menu that includes at least one dairy serving from the calcium-rich group, and at least one meat serving from the protein-rich group.

℗ Women who do not eat beef, fish, or chicken, will need to obtain vitamin B_{12} from a supplement or consume enough dairy, eggs, or enriched grains to meet the RDA. Each cup of yogurt or milk carries 1.0 mcg.; one ounce of cheese, 0.2 mcg.; one egg, 0.6 mcg.; and each serving of enriched ready-to-eat cereal, 1.5 mcg.

Calcium

RDA: Adult women 1,000 mg., pregnant women under age 18, 1,300 mg.; over age 19, 1,000 mg.

Calcium is an essential nutrient during pregnancy because it is needed to build strong bones and to form teeth that will emerge after birth. It is also needed by muscles and nerves, and is necessary for initiating blood clotting and regulating blood pressure.

Because this nutrient is so important, during pregnancy changes in calcium-regulating hormones occur that make calcium absorption and reabsorption from the kidneys and intestines more efficient. These changes allow the baby to receive the calcium it needs for developing bones and teeth, while the mother's blood and bone calcium supply is protected for her own use. (Although research suggests that, despite the increased efficiency of calcium absorption, some calcium may still be withdrawn from the mother's bones.)

Women consuming below 600 mg. of calcium will develop a negative calcium balance, meaning their intake does not keep pace with their needs. The woman who eats only one small calcium source per day is probably below 600 mg.

An inverse relationship has been seen between calcium intake and high blood pressure. Some studies have demonstrated that calcium can reduce the incidence of pregnancy-induced high blood pressure, a potentially life-threatening condition (see page 149). However, large doses of calcium to treat pregnancy-induced high blood pressure should not be taken unless recommended by your health-care provider.

Calcium has long been credited as a treatment for leg cramps, but in one study when 2,000 mg. of calcium was given daily for three weeks there was no improvement in the incidence of leg cramps as compared to a group given a placebo.

Supplementation at levels much above the RDA are not recommended. A high intake of calcium may lead to constipation and may interfere with the absorption of both iron and zinc. The National Academy of Sciences has set an Upper Tolerable Intake Level (UL) of 2,500 mg. a day.

Good calcium sources: All dairy foods including milk, cheese, and yogurt. Fish with edible bones such as canned salmon and sardines. Tofu processed with calcium sulfate. Vegetables including broccoli, kale, collards, mustard greens, turnip greens. Foods or mixed dishes made with milk or cheese, including puddings and casseroles.

Recommendations to meet your calcium needs:

◎ Eat the recommended servings from the calcium-rich group. Each serving of dairy foods carries approximately 300 mg. of calcium.

◎ If you are lactose intolerant use low-lactose calcium-rich foods such as lactose-free milk and cottage cheese. Yogurt and aged cheese are often well tolerated by people with lactose intolerance. Vegetable sources of calcium carry no lactose.

⊚   A supplement may be required if a mother is not able to eat the recommended number of calcium containing foods.

Magnesium

RDA: Adult women 310 mg.; pregnant women under age 18, 400 mg.; over age 19, 350 mg.

Magnesium is needed for the metabolism of carbohydrate, protein, and fat. It also assists in the health and function of the intestines, bones, and kidneys.

Food surveys suggest that pregnant women get less magnesium than the RDA, but deficiencies do not occur because the RDA has been established with a generous margin of error. However, a lower frequency of fetal-growth retardation and preeclampsia has been seen when women take supplements of magnesium. Also, one study has found supplemental magnesium to be effective in treating pregnancy-induced leg cramps. There is not enough data to recommend routine magnesium supplementation during pregnancy, but it is advisable for women to eat foods that are rich in this nutrient.

Good magnesium sources: nuts, seeds, dry beans, whole grains, scallops, and oysters. Spinach, beet greens, and broccoli contain small amounts.

Recommendations to meet your magnesium needs:

⊚   Use seeds or nuts on salads or to top vegetable dishes. One ounce of sunflower seeds carries 100 mg. of magnesium.

⊚ Eat at least three whole-grain foods daily. Half a cup of raw brown rice carries 131 mg. of magnesium, whereas white rice carries only 23 mg. Try quinoa, a whole grain that cooks like white rice. Half a cup raw carries 178 mg. of magnesium, and it's a good calcium source, too. One tablespoon of wheat germ contains 20 mg. of magnesium.

Iron

RDA: Adult women 15 mg.; pregnant women 30 mg.

Iron is the mineral essential for the production of hemoglobin. Hemoglobin carries oxygen from the lungs to the tissues, and it is used to make enzymes that the body relies upon to produce energy. In the first trimester of pregnancy the demand for iron is not great, in part because the cessation of menstruation brings about a natural conservation of the nutrient. In the second and third trimester, however, the demand for iron increases. Pregnant women need more iron to supply the growing baby and placenta and to meet the iron demands created by an increase in red-blood-cell mass.

To detect iron deficiency anemia, most women will have their iron levels checked at their first doctor's visit. This is done by measuring hemoglobin and hematocrit blood levels. Read more about iron deficiency anemia on page 141. An iron supplement is often advised, beginning at the twelfth week of pregnancy.

Good iron sources: Meat, including beef, lamb, and pork, eggs, vegetables, fortified cereals. Animal-source (heme) iron from meats provides a very absorbable form of iron.

Plant-source (nonheme) iron is also good, but is not as well absorbed as the iron in meat-based foods.

Recommendations to meet your iron needs:

ᪧ Vitamin C enhances iron absorption. Pregnant women are advised to eat a source of vitamin C with every meal. Try orange juice or sliced fruit at breakfast, sliced tomato at lunch, and a baked potato or fresh green salad at dinner.

ᪧ Eat at least one iron-rich serving from the protein-rich group every day.

ᪧ Tea, calcium phosphate (found in supplements), bran, and antacids can interfere with the nonheme forms of iron found in plant foods. For this reason, don't consume any of these with your meals.

ᪧ Take iron supplements between meals with liquids other than milk, tea, or coffee. Citrus juice, vegetable juice, or water are better choices.

Zinc

RDA: Adult women 12 mg.; pregnant women 15 mg.

Zinc is a very important nutrient involved in protein metabolism and in the fundamental process of cell division. Low blood levels of zinc during pregnancy may be associated with pregnancy-induced hypertension, prolonged labor, excessive bleeding, and impaired growth of the baby.

During pregnancy women appear to consume in the range of 8.8 to 14.4 mg. per day. Among vegetarian women the intake could be lower. A special concern is the possibility that iron supplements can lower the level of zinc in the mother's blood. The Institute of Medicine's report, *Nutrition During Pregnancy*, recommends that pregnant women taking more than 30 mg. of supplemental iron should take small amounts of zinc to compensate for the negative effect iron can have on zinc absorption. It is only the supplemental form of iron that interferes with zinc. Food sources of iron do not.

Seventy percent of the zinc we consume comes from animal sources. Whole-grain foods carry a less absorbable form of zinc as well as fiber and phytate, which can interfere with zinc absorption.

Good zinc sources: Meat, liver, eggs, and seafood.

Recommendations to meet your zinc needs:

✆ Make at least one of your daily protein-rich choices an animal source such as eggs or meat. One egg carries .72 mg. of zinc, most of it in the yolk; 4 ounces of ground turkey contains 4 mg., and the same amount of ground beef contains just over 5 mg.

✆ The Institute of Medicine recommends that women taking over 60 mg. of iron to treat iron deficiency anemia should take a multivitamin/mineral that carries 15 mg. of zinc.

Iodine

RDA: Adult women 150 mcg.; pregnant women 175 mcg.

Iodine is an essential component of the thyroid hormones. The incidence of iodine deficiency in the United

States dropped dramatically after iodized salt was introduced to our food supply in 1924. This has significant health consequences because a pregnant woman who is unable to get enough iodine could have a child with growth abnormalities and neurological complications. The most familiar consequence of iodine deficiency is goiter, a condition in which the thyroid gland grows to an abnormal size. In countries where iodine intake is low, such as Asia, Africa, South America, and Europe, iodine deficiency can be a serious public health issue.

Good iodine sources: Seafood is the best source and, of course, iodized salt.

Recommendations to meet iodine needs: No special effort needs to be made to meet the iodine requirement. Normal salt intake in cooking and in prepared foods should be sufficient.

Selenium

RDA: Adult women 55 mcg.; pregnant women 65 mcg.

Selenium is a trace mineral that works like vitamin E to protect the body from damage by binding with free radicals. Selenium deficiencies have been documented in areas such as China where the soil was deficient or in severely ill people on inadequate feeding programs. Food surveys find that pregnant women consume about 70 mcg. of this nutrient, which is an adequate amount.

There is no need for pregnant women to take supplements. When consumed at excessive levels (30 mg.), toxicity can occur.

Good selenium sources: Seafood, kidneys, liver, and most

meats. Grains and seeds vary in their content, and fruits and vegetables generally contain little of this nutrient.

Recommendations to meet your selenium needs: The requirement for selenium should be easily obtained if a woman chooses a variety of foods from each food group.

Vitamin A

RDA: 800 mcg.; there is no increase in the RDA during pregnancy.

Vitamin A is best known for its contribution to vision, but it is also essential to the growth and reproduction of healthy cells and to our immune system. Vitamin A comes in two forms: the preformed retenoid, found in animal products, and the carotenoid or plant form, most familiar to us as beta carotene.

Vitamin A deficiency can cause blindness, but in the United States this is uncommon because most Americans get what they need from food. The RDA for vitamin A does not increase during pregnancy, not because it is unimportant but because women eat adequate amounts in food and can store vitamin A in the liver.

Do not take high doses of vitamin A, as it can cause headaches, vomiting, hair loss, and liver damage. Women taking very large doses in the first trimester of their pregnancy have an increased incidence of spontaneous abortion and birth defects. Some acne medications may contain high doses of preformed vitamin A. Ask your doctor about the use of all medications. Signs of toxicity occur only with sustained daily intakes of supplements that are consumed at very high dosages, such as ten times the RDA, or when large amounts of fish liver or fish liver oils rich in vitamin A are consumed routinely. Routine supplementation is not recommended.

Good vitamin A sources: While the richest sources include liver and fish liver oils, other good sources include fortified milk, eggs, carrots, dark green leafy vegetables, and vegetable-based soups.

Recommendations to meet your vitamin A needs:

◎ Eat one dark green or *dark orange fruit* or vegetable every day.

◎ Eat three or more servings of fruit daily.

◎ Eat two or more servings of vegetables daily.

◎ Drink vitamin A–fortified milk.

Vitamin D

RDA: Adult women 5 mcg.; RDA does not increase in pregnancy.

Vitamin D is the nutrient that works with calcium to make strong bones and a healthy skeleton. When intake is poor, bones are not properly mineralized and rickets can occur. Early in the twentieth century, it was discovered that rickets could be prevented and cured in children if they were exposed to the sun. The sunlight creates a supply of vitamin D by synthesizing the nutrient from natural precursors in the skin. Because sun exposure is not always adequate and deficiencies can be damaging, vitamin D is added to all commercial milk, making rickets rare in the United States. Vitamin D deficiency is not uncommon among women in Europe, where milk is not routinely fortified with vitamin D.

It is the amount of exposure to sunlight that determines our need for vitamin D. A low vitamin D intake from food, combined with low sun exposure, results in low blood levels in the mother and in the blood of the umbilical cord. A child born to a mother with a vitamin D deficiency can have low blood-calcium levels that cause neuromuscular problems. Despite the importance of vitamin D, routine supplementation is not recommended during pregnancy. Vitamin D supplements consumed in combination with vitamin D–fortified milk can add up to toxic levels. The National Academy of Sciences has set a UL for vitamin D of 2,000 IU or 50 mg. a day.

Good vitamin D sources: Vitamin D–fortified milk is a major food source. One quart carries 10 mcg. Eggs, butter, and fortified margarine are also good sources.

Recommendations to meet your vitamin D needs:

◎ Women who avoid drinking milk and live in a climate that limits exposure to the sun may need to take a supplement of 10 mcg. of vitamin D per day to meet their need. Discuss this with your doctor.

◎ Drink and cook with vitamin D–fortified milk.

◎ Take a morning and evening stroll to increase sun exposure.

◎ Use small amounts of real butter or fortified margarine for cooking and eating.

Vitamin K

RDA: Adult women 65 mcg.; there is no increase in the RDA while pregnant.

Vitamin K is a fat-soluble vitamin that is best known for its contribution to blood clotting. We obtain vitamin K from food, and some is made in the intestine. Most women eat in the range of 300 to 500 mcg. per day. Since our intake greatly exceeds the RDA, there is no increase recommended during pregnancy.

Vitamin K deficiencies can occur, but they are limited to people who have a serious malabsorption problem or require long-term treatment with antibiotics. Antibiotics, when they are taken for long periods, can harm the intestinal bacteria that make some of the vitamin K we need. Women who have a malabsorption condition or are on long-term antibiotic therapy may need a vitamin K supplement.

When your baby is born he does not have a supply of vitamin K to protect him from blood hemorrhage. At birth, all infants receive a one-time injection of vitamin K to take care of this early bleeding risk.

Good vitamin K sources: Vitamin K is present in a wide variety of foods, especially leafy vegetables, brussels sprouts, cabbage, dairy foods, meat, eggs, fruit, and liver.

Recommendations to meet vitamin K needs:

◎ Eat two or more vegetables daily. Make one of them a green leafy choice such as kale or dark green lettuce.

◎ Take supplements only on the advice of your physician. Short-term antibiotic therapy should not impact on vitamin K.

ADDITIONAL IMPORTANT NUTRIENTS IN FOODS

The nutrients biotin, pantothenic acid, copper, manganese, fluoride, chromium, and molybdenum are all nutrients recognized to be essential in all stages of life. However there is not enough information available on these nutrients to make specific recommendations during pregnancy. Instead the National Research Council has created estimated safe and adequate daily dietary intakes. The recommended intakes for adults precedes the description for each of these nutrients.

Biotin

Estimated safe and adequate daily dietary intake: 30 mcg.

Biotin is a vitamin and coenzyme for several important reactions such as the metabolism of fat, carbohydrates, and proteins. Biotin deficiencies have not been reported except under experimental situations. Biotin is available in food and can be made in the intestines, making a biotin deficiency unlikely.

Good biotin sources include: Liver, egg yolk, soy flour, cereals, and yeast. Fruit and meat are poor sources.

Pantothenic Acid

Estimated safe and adequate daily dietary intakes: Adult women 5 mg.; pregnant women 6 mg.

Pantothenic acid is a member of the B complex group of vitamins and a component in energy production. Deficiencies of this nutrient are virtually unknown because it is distributed widely in a variety of foods and it may even be produced in the intestine.

Good pantothenic acid sources: animal meats, whole-grain cereals, and legumes. Milk, vegetables, and fruit carry small amounts.

Copper

Estimated safe and adequate daily dietary intakes: 1.5– 3.0 mg.

Copper plays a key role in enzymes that are important to proper metabolism, the development of connective tissue, iron utilization, and wound healing. Copper deficiencies caused by diet have not been seen in pregnant women, and food surveys suggest that women consume 1.4 to 1.8 mg. per day while pregnant. Zinc supplements in the 50 mg. range can interfere with copper metabolism and absorption. The Institute of Medicine, in its report *Nutrition During Pregnancy,* recommends that supplemental zinc should be given in combination with 2 mg. of copper to compensate for the poor absorption that will occur when copper is given with zinc.

Good copper sources: Liver, seafood, nuts, and seeds.

Manganese

Estimated safe and adequate daily dietary intakes: 2.0– 5.0 mg.

Manganese makes up part of two enzymes that are essential to our health. Manganese deficiencies are virtually unknown. Some data suggest that iron supplements may interfere with manganese absorption, but not enough is known to routinely advise its use during pregnancy.

Good manganese sources: whole grains, cereal products, fruit, vegetables, and tea. Dairy products, meat, fish, and poultry are poor sources.

Fluoride

Estimated safe and adequate daily dietary intakes: 3.0 mg. for adult women and pregnant women over age 19.

Fluoride protects against cavities by accumulating in the exterior layer of the tooth enamel to make it hard. When women take fluoride during pregnancy a decrease in cavities has been reported in their babies. However, not enough evidence exists to recommend fluoride supplementation while pregnant, and excessive fluoride can lead to discoloration of teeth.

Good fluoride sources: Tea and some marine fish consumed with the bones. Cow's milk is a poor source.

Chromium

Estimated safe and adequate daily dietary intakes: 50– 200 mcg.

Chromium is a component of the substance known as glucose tolerance factor (GTF), which works with insulin, the hormone responsible for controlling blood sugar. Abnormal blood-sugar levels can result from a very low chromium intake. Chromium picolinate is an easily digested form of chromium that is currently being marketed as a weight-loss aid. However, there is no evidence that it accelerates fat loss or curbs appetite as its supporters suggest.

Good chromium sources: brewer's yeast, liver, meat, peanut butter, whole grains, oysters, and nuts.

Molybdenum

Estimated safe and adequate daily dietary intake: 75–250 mcg.

Molybdenum is a component of several important enzymes. It is needed in very small amounts and deficiencies are unknown. Adults usually eat about 76 to 109 mcg. per day and it is easy to meet the recommended estimates. Molybdenum supplements are not necessary during pregnancy.

Good molybdenum sources: milk, beans, breads, and cereals.

Regardless of how you feel about weight gain and pregnancy, nutrition and eating well are essential to your well-being and that of your baby. Use this section and refer to it as often as needed to answer questions about food, supplements, and managing the symptoms that can develop during pregnancy.

3

How Much Is Enough?

Any woman concerned about gaining too much weight during pregnancy would probably like to hear a nutritionist tell her exactly how many calories and grams of fat her body needs to grow a healthy baby and prevent excessive fat gain. In truth, we can't predict calorie needs with absolute precision. Once a woman becomes pregnant, biological changes unique to pregnancy affect her need for calories and even determine how her body will gain weight. We can, however, make some reasonable estimates that can keep both mother and baby well nourished.

The reason it is difficult to be precise about caloric needs is that the human body uses calories differently when pregnant. For example, research studies reveal that a woman's resting metabolism, the rate at which she burns calories, increases during pregnancy. The degree of change in resting metabolism is highly variable, but it does exist and can have a major effect on caloric needs. Some studies have also found a change in dietary thermogenesis in pregnant women. Dietary thermogenesis is the energy expended to complete the tasks of digestion, absorption, transportation, and storage of nutrients after a meal is eaten. When the thermic effect of eating was measured during pregnancy in seven first-time mothers it was found that their thermic response was reduced by 28 percent in midpregnancy and 15 percent in the late pregnancy. A reduction in a pregnant woman's thermic response to meals could be a way that her body conserves calories.

The extra weight a woman gains when pregnant will increase her need for calories. For example, a woman who weighs 140 pounds at conception and 155 pounds in her second trimester should need more calories to perform the routine activities of daily life. Then again, the extra weight of the developing pregnancy may cause a woman to be less active, reducing her calorie needs. Changes in lifestyle will affect energy needs as well. The woman who gives up her full-time job may be less active at home and find she snacks more just because she has more contact with food. All of these are variables that are hard to assess. What we do know unequivocally is that you need to eat more when you are pregnant, although exactly how much is uncertain.

First and foremost, your goal when pregnant is to keep yourself well nourished. One of the best unplanned opportunities to study the effect of calorie restriction on women during pregnancy occurred during the Dutch famine of World War II. Due to a food shortage, and strict rationing for a six-month period, Dutch women experienced a gradual decrease in the amount of food available to them until it reached a low point of less than 1,500 calories per day. This deprivation was followed by a rapid reintroduction of available calories, up to 3,200 calories per day. At the height of the famine, the average infant birth weight was much lower than it was previous to the famine and birth weight rebounded in the babies born to mothers after the famine. This unplanned restriction of calories during pregnancy showed that women deprived of adequate calories delivered babies that weighed significantly less than they should, putting their children at risk for medical complications.

WHAT IS THE RIGHT AMOUNT?

In the United States, the National Research Council has established the caloric needs of pregnant women to be 2,500 calories. This is calculated by adding 300 additional calories to the 2,200 calories needed by nonpregnant women of childbearing age.

This 300 calorie increase has been determined based on the theoretical calorie cost of a pregnancy. It is estimated that over the course of pregnancy the body will need a total of 55,000 calories. A woman can easily meet this 300 calorie increase by adding a glass of milk and a small muffin; a bowl of cereal and milk with fruit; or a yogurt and a few graham crackers to her menu. (In the first trimester, when growth and weight gain are gradual, a woman needs only 100 additional calories per day.) Remember: when adding calories, make your food additions nutritious ones.

To meet your need for key nutrients it is essential to look at your total diet and address any nutritional problems you may have. It is quite possible to eat a 2,500 calorie diet and have half the calories come from nutrient-poor foods. In the first 13 weeks of pregnancy a woman will want to consume around 2,300 calories a day. Women of short stature may need less, while very tall women will need more. Women who are underweight will want to move right up to the 2,500 calorie plan. Don't focus on calories alone. Nutritionists use calories as a starting point. Pay attention to the number of servings you need from each food group suggested below, and you will automatically consume the proper balance of calories and nutrients. Examine eating habits you may have that are not ideal, such as skipping breakfast, having a light lunch with soda or dessert, a donut at 3:00, a large high-fat dinner, or consuming salty, processed snacks at night. Don't count calories, but instead monitor weight progress and diet quality. Eat at least the minimum amounts from the food groups below to get the essential nutrients you need in the first weeks of pregnancy. A complete list of serving sizes for each food group follows on pages 74–81.

In the first 13 weeks:

FOOD GROUP	RECOMMENDED SERVING PER DAY
Bread/starch	7+
Calcium-rich	3–4
Protein-rich	2–3
Vegetable	2–4
Fruit	3–5
Fat	3+

After the first 13 weeks, to reach 2,500 calories increase your food intake to:

Bread/starch	11
Calcium-rich	3–4
Protein-rich	2–3
Vegetable	4
Fruit	6
Fat	3–7

Wow! This Is Way Too Much Food!

Twenty-five-hundred calories is an amount of food that will keep a normal-weight woman well nourished and help her gain the recommended 25 to 35 pounds required. Although when you look at the amount of recommended food it can seem excessive, the serving sizes nutritionists use are in most cases actually smaller than what is customary. For example, a 12-ounce container of juice actually counts as three servings of fruit and a 2-cup portion of pasta counts as four servings from the starch/bread group. A serving of steak is about 3 to 4 ounces, not the 12 ounces commonly served at most restaurants. In other cases, food choices can be much denser in calories. For example, a croissant containing 400-plus calories should count as three or four servings from the bread/starch group, not one. This food plan emphasizes lots of fruits and vegetables rich in fiber and nutrients, which is more than most people are accustomed to. More of these foods are added to help women meet their need for nutrition and fiber, and to keep the ratio of fat in the diet to approximately 30 percent.

Exactly How Much Fat Do I Need?

Many women eat very-low-fat diets to keep weight down. There are no established fat recommendations for pregnancy, but a reasonable goal is 30 percent of calories. This amount is recommended for the population as a whole and is appropriate for pregnant women too. Thirty percent of 2,500 calories is approximately 85 grams of fat per day. Women who eat only 20 percent of their calories as fat may find it difficult to meet their energy needs while pregnant.

Women need some fat and should eat the foods that naturally carry it, such as cooking oils, butter, margarine, meat, fish, poultry, and whole-wheat and prepared grain products such as bread or muffins. Many of these foods are good sources of nutrients such as vitamin E and essential fatty acids. And as a bonus, fats added to food and used in cooking also enhance flavor.

Most of the fat you consume will come from the protein-rich food group, and obviously from the fat group. The three to seven recommended servings from the fat group are not set amounts that you must strive for. These recommendations are suggestions to help you read labels and budget the amounts of added fat servings you use on food. Many of these fat servings will be consumed in combination with foods from the bread/starch group. Start reading labels and you will find that a homemade muffin carries 5 grams of fat or one fat serving, and a bowl of granola-type cereal carries at least one serving of hidden fat. Read more about this on page 79 under the Fat Group heading.

One Day's Menu

This menu is an example of a 2,500-calorie day. Use it as a guide and learning tool to see which foods fit in the various food groups.

Food Group	Amount	Sample Food
BREAKFAST		
Calcium-rich	1	1 cup low-fat milk
Fruit	2	8 oz. orange juice
Bread/starch	3	1 sl. toast and 1½ cup ready-to-eat cereal
Fat	1	1 tsp. butter
Free	NA	coffee/tea (without milk or sugar)
MIDMORNING SNACK		
Calcium-rich	1	1 cup yogurt
Bread/starch	1	⅓ cup wheat germ

LUNCH

Calcium-rich	1	1 cup milk
Protein-rich	1	3 oz. sliced chicken
Bread/starch	2	1 roll
Vegetable	2	1 tomato, sliced; 1 cup salad
Fat	3	2 tsp. mayonnaise; 1 tbsp. salad dressing

MIDAFTERNOON SNACK

Protein-rich	⅓	1 tbsp. peanut butter
Bread/starch	1	3 graham crackers
Fruit	2	1 cup grapefruit juice

SUPPER

Calcium-rich	½	½ cup lowfat milk
Protein-rich	1	4 ounces cooked steak
Vegetable	2	½ cup carrots ½ cup green beans
Bread/starch	3	1½ cup noodles
Fat	3	3 tsp. butter
Fruit	1	1 peach

EVENING SNACK

| Calcium-rich | ½ | ½ cup milk |
| Bread/starch | 1 | ¾ cup cereal |

ESTABLISH A WEIGHT GOAL

With the help of your doctor, establish weight goals for the total pregnancy and each trimester. As explained in Chapter 2, the Institute of Medicine recommends a gradual weight gain of 25 to 35 pounds for women with a normal body mass index (BMI). The weight gain in the first trimester should be small, ranging from two to five pounds, depending on BMI. From week 14 to 40 the rate of weight gain should be slow and steady, about one pound per week. Women who gain less than two pounds per month need to look carefully at their diet, as do women who are gaining more than six and a half pounds per month.

The purpose of setting a weight goal with your doctor is to make yourself aware of what is safe and healthy for you and to help monitor your progress. Since some women actually fear gaining weight, it can be helpful to know what is considered a normal weight gain. Use the goals you set to support your eating decisions. Keep in mind that your body is not a machine. Women almost never gain weight in a completely consistent, even fashion. Focus on healthy eating, and strive for a slow and steady gain without any sudden shifts. Your growing child needs nutrients all the time to develop best, and large swings in weight can indicate poor nutrition or fluid retention.

Use the recommended serving suggestions for each food group on page 63 and the one-day food menu on page 65 to help you meet your need for calories and nutrition. If your weight is progressing to meet the goals you established with your doctor, all you have to do is "eat to appetite," (that is, as your appetite dictates) making sure you eat at least the minimum recommended number of servings from each food group. Try to eat a wide variety of food. The more varied your menu, the more balanced your nutrient intake will be.

If you find you are gaining too fast or not fast enough, try a more individualized plan based on height and activity. Many women who are gaining too fast may find that increased activity such as a daily walk will be better than decreased food. Read about exercise in Chapter 6 and talk to your doctor about the role exercise can play in your pregnancy. Unlike weight gain, exercise is a factor you can control and for women it is one of the key components to weight control and good health during and after pregnancy. (Being fit may also make delivery easier to deal with.)

HOW TO CREATE A MORE INDIVIDUALIZED EATING PLAN

If you use the 2,500-calorie meal plan but require a more individualized approach, use the calorie determination system described below. These are only rough calculations; outside of a research lab caloric estimates are only educated guesses. Nevertheless, these estimations can help you adjust your food intake to meet your determined calorie needs.

Estimating Your Calorie Needs

First determine your nonpregnant ideal body weight (IBW). For many women their weight at age 21 is often their IBW, or use the following:

Allow 100 pounds for the first five feet of height, plus five pounds for each additional inch. (Small-frame women can subtract 10 percent and large-frame women can add 10 percent to the total.)

For example, the IBW for a medium frame 5'8" woman would be 140 pounds.

To double-check the accuracy of your IBW, use the BMI chart in Chapter 1. Based on your height, your IBW should be between 20 and 26 on the BMI chart. A nonpregnant weight range for a 5'8" tall woman would be between 131 to 171 pounds.

Your estimated nonpregnant IBW _____.

Next, multiply your nonpregnant ideal body weight by the activity number below that matches your exercise habits. Most of us fall into the sedentary category unless we engage in substantial regular exercise. Women who exercise to sweat, 20 to 30 minutes three times a week, are engaging in moderate exercise. If you are less active, count yourself in the sedentary group. Read more about exercise and pregnancy in Chapter 6.

13 for sedentary activity: some walking, typing, sewing, ironing, cooking, seated and standing activities, light housekeeping.

15 for moderate activity: walking briskly, weeding, hoeing, carrying loads, bicycling, tennis, dancing.

20 for heavy activity: jogging, heavy manual labor, climbing, digging.

Your daily calorie requirement when not pregnant is (IBW × activity number) = _____.

Finally, add the 300 additional calories recommended during pregnancy by the National Research Council to this total.

Your daily total calorie requirement when pregnant is:_____

For example, our theoretical mother who is 5'8" and sedentary has an IBW of 140 pounds and a calorie requirement of 1,820 when not pregnant and 2,120 calories when pregnant. If she is moderately active, her calorie needs are 2,100 when not pregnant and 2,400 while pregnant. If she were very active, she would need 2,800 when not pregnant and 3,100 while pregnant.

You can see that some women may need significantly more or less than the 2,500 calories recommended by the RDA. It is not recommended that any pregnant woman go below 1,800 calories per day.

Once you have calculated an individualized calorie level, use it to select the number of servings from each food group to meet this level. Always eat the minimum number of servings from each food group so you consume adequate calcium, protein, and iron, and make sure you are gaining weight at the level recommended by your doctor.

FOOD GROUP	SERVINGS PER DAY
1800–2000 calories	
Calcium-rich group	3
Protein-rich	2
Bread/starch	8–9
Vegetable	3–4
Fruit	3
Fat	3–5
2,100–2,300	
Calcium-rich	3–4
Protein-rich	2
Bread/starch	9–10
Vegetable	3–4
Fruit	3–4
Fat	6–7

2,400–2,600

Calcium-rich	3–4
Protein-rich	2–3
Bread/starch	10–12
Vegetable	4
Fruit	5
Fat	7

2,700–3,000

Calcium-rich	4
Protein-rich	2–3
Bread/starch	12–15
Vegetable	5–6
Fruit	5–6
Fat	7–8

Multiple Births

The mother who is carrying more than one child will obviously need more calories. Women often don't learn about a multiple birth until their pregnancy has progressed. Mothers of twins may restrict their weight gain if they do not know until late in their pregnancy that they are carrying twins. This may explain why in 1986, when researchers looked at birth weights of babies, less than 2 percent of the births were twins, yet 16 percent of the low birth weight infants were twins. Anemia may be more common in mothers of twins, too. Extra nutrition and calories are important for these women, which is why women carrying twins are advised to gain more weight, a total of 35 to 45 pounds, or about one and a half pounds per week during the second and third trimester.

Any Questions?

What if I was underweight before I became pregnant? With the help of your doctor, establish a weight-gain goal for the first 13 weeks of pregnancy. Most women don't need to worry about eating more until after the thirteenth week, but women who are underweight at conception should eat an additional 300 calories of food beginning in the first trimester. When calculating your calorie needs as shown on page 68, be sure to use ideal body weight as defined there rather than your actual weight or what you think is your IBW. Then strive to meet your doctor's weight-gain goal or the recommended weight-gain goals established by the Institute of Medicine of two to five pounds in the first trimester and at least one pound each week thereafter.

What if I was overweight before I became pregnant? Focus on the quality of your diet, eat the recommended amounts from each food group, but don't add any extra food right away. Ask your doctor about an appropriate weight gain. In the second and third trimester a weight gain of less than two-thirds of a pound per week, or three to four pounds per month is usually advised for a woman who is overweight at conception. A total weight gain of 15 to 25 pounds is recommended by the Institute of Medicine for women with a high BMI, less if you would be classified as obese (BMI greater than 29). (See Chapter 1 for BMI calculation chart.)

What if I am gaining weight too fast? First, talk it over with your health-care provider. Weight measurements can be inaccurate and not a true indicator of fat gain. All sorts of things can cause weight to fluctuate and most of them have nothing to do with the health of your pregnancy. However, look at the trend. If several weight checks show that you are gaining more than a pound a week or more than six and a half pounds per month, you should look at how and what you are eating. To help you identify food problems, keep a food record as described on page 85. Also, discuss the need for additional, gentle exercise with your doctor.

What if I am frustrated with the amount I am gaining? For some women it can be impossible to identify how they might gain more than their goal weight. In this case, seek out professional help. Contact a registered dietitian. In most cases, a trained nutritionist will complete a nutrition history with you and give you the individual care and counseling you need. In many cases, a trained professional can identify an eating problem that may not be obvious to you.

PUTTING THE PLAN INTO ACTION—THE NINE FOOD GROUPS

Good nutrition is the most important tenet of any food plan while pregnant. First, determine the number of servings you need to eat from each of the six primary food groups. (Refer to page 68 where you calculated your calorie needs.) In addition to the six food groups there are three additional groups: the Free list, the Combination list, and a list of foods to eat only once a day. I call this last group the Daily Option list. Foods in these groups add flavor and variety, but they often do not contain the nutrients required during pregnancy.

For good nutrition, eat the minimum number of servings from each food group daily, and for adequate calories, eat the recommended number of servings. These recommended servings add up to a 2,500-calorie intake, which is an amount

appropriate for most pregnant women. If you have calculated an individualized plan that puts you at a calorie level
below or above the 2,500 calories recommended, make the
appropriate adjustments by writing your serving size above
each food group.

Always eat the minimum number of recommended servings from each group. If you do this, you will insure
adequate intake of protein and calcium, nutrients that are
very important when pregnant.

Bread/Starch Group

Foods in this group are rich in carbohydrate and low in fat.
They are good sources of thiamin, niacin, and iron, and
should be a major part of your menu. Whole-grain foods are
good sources of fiber, so try to eat three servings of whole-
grain foods daily, such as whole-wheat bread or cereal, or
brown rice. Bran cereals are a good source of zinc.

Each serving in this group will carry approximately 80 to
100 calories, 15 grams of carbohydrate, 3 grams of protein,
and up to 2 grams of fat. When labels indicate that a food
carries 5 or more grams of fat per serving, count it as one of
your fat servings.

Minimum daily amount   *7 servings*
Recommended daily amount   *11 servings*

A serving is:

1 slice of bread
½ cup cooked rice or pasta
½ cup cooked cereal

1 ounce (about ¾ cup) ready-to-eat cereal

½ bagel or English muffin

1 4-inch pancake, 1 waffle, or 1 slice French toast

1 8-inch soft tortilla

1 small pita pocket

Snack Foods in the Bread/Starch Group

This includes all foods made from grain including: bread sticks, biscuits, cookies, crackers, popcorn, cake, and cupcakes. To determine the size of an 80 to 100 calorie portion, read the Nutrition Facts Panel that accompanies the product. The serving size will vary from product to product. When reading labels, pay close attention to fat. A 5-gram portion of fat is equal to one serving from the fat group or 1 teaspoon of butter.

Calcium-rich Group

The foods included in this group provide approximately 300 mg. of calcium, 100 calories, 12 grams of carbohydrate, 8 grams of protein, and 2.5 grams of fat per serving. They are also a rich source of vitamin D and riboflavin. Nonfat and low-fat milks are recommended over whole milk because they are equal in nutrition but have far fewer fat calories.

Minimum daily amount   *3 servings*
Recommended daily amount   *3–4 servings*

A serving is:

1 cup milk or yogurt

1½–2 oz. cheese

Nondairy Calcium-rich Foods

The following foods carry 300 mg. of calcium per serving, the same amount as in milk. Some foods listed below carry fewer calories and protein than dairy sources of calcium. This can be significant for women who are underweight or unable to eat the recommended number of servings from the protein-rich group. Most are not fortified with vitamins A and D.

8 oz. tofu (172 calories, 18 grams protein)

1½ cups cooked greens* (50–60 calories, 8 grams protein)

1 cup fortified soy milk† (80 calories, 7 grams protein)

1 cup calcium fortified rice milk† (130 calories, 1 gram protein)

1 cup goat's milk (168 calories, 9 grams protein)

1 cup kefir (160 calories, 9 grams protein)

Protein-rich Group

A serving from this food group will carry approximately 165 to 225 calories, 21 grams of protein, and 9 to 15 grams of fat. Good sources of iron are indicated with an asterisk.

---

*Collards, beet greens, and spinach may contain significant amounts of oxalic acid, which can potentially interfere with calcium absorption.
†Soy and rice milk look and taste similar to cow's milk but they are extremely low in calcium unless fortified. Rice milk carries only 1 gram of protein per cup. On food labels, the Nutrition Facts Panel will list calcium as a percentage. A food carrying 30 percent of the required calcium per serving is a superb source of calcium.

Minimum daily amount   *2 servings*
Recommended daily amount   *2–3 servings*

A serving is:

3 oz. cooked lean, beef, veal, pork, poultry or fish*

¾ cup flaked fish such as tuna, salmon, or crab*

¾ cup cottage or ricotta cheese (cheese carries both protein and calcium, which is why it appears in both the protein-rich and calcium-rich food groups)

3 oz. hard cheese

3 oz. sliced low-fat deli meats

1½ cup cooked beans‡

1 egg or 2 tbsp. of peanut butter counts as 1 ounce of lean meat or ⅓ serving

    Regular cheese, sausage, cold cuts, and hot dogs are high-fat foods that are best limited to once per week. Low-fat substitutes are available in most stores and carry protein equal to their high-fat counterparts.

Vegetable Group

The foods within this list provide approximately 25 calories per serving. They also contain 5 grams of carbohydrate, 2

---

‡Baked beans contain about 8 grams of protein and 175 calories in a half-cup portion.

grams of protein, and are good sources of vitamin A and vitamin C as well as fiber. Choose a dark green, leafy, or orange vegetable three or four times a week.

Minimum daily amount   *2 servings*
Recommended daily amount   *4 servings*

A serving portion is:

½ cup chopped or cooked vegetable or juice
1 cup raw leafy vegetable

   Good vegetable choices include: asparagus, bean sprouts, green and wax beans, beets, broccoli, brussels sprouts, cabbage, carrots, cauliflower, corn, eggplant, greens, kohlrabi, leeks, mushrooms, okra, onions, peas, pea pods, peppers (all colors), potatoes, rutabaga, sauerkraut, spinach, squash, tomatoes, tomato juice, carrot juice, turnips, yellow squash, zucchini.

Fruit Group

Each serving provides approximately 60 calories and 15 grams of carbohydrate. These foods are a rich source of fiber and vitamin C.

Minimum daily amount   *3 servings*
Recommended daily amount   *6 servings*

A serving is:

1 piece of fruit (apple, kiwi, nectarine, peach, pear, tangerine, orange, small banana)

½ cup juice (select real fruit juice such as apple, orange, and grapefruit)

¼ cup dried fruit

½ cup canned or chopped fruit

Fat Group

Foods in this group contain approximately 5 grams of fat per serving and 45 calories. They carry no protein or carbohydrate but they are often a good source of vitamin E and, most important, they add flavor to food.

Minimum daily amount   *3 servings*
The recommended daily amount   *3–7§ servings*

A serving is:

1 tsp. margarine, mayonnaise, butter and all cooking oils

1 tbsp. cream, cream cheese, or salad dressing.

---

§The recommended seven servings is not an amount you *must* strive for. It is an amount of fat that is easily consumed in the course of eating a healthful diet. For example, if you add a teaspoon of butter to your toast at breakfast, a teaspoon of mayonnaise in a sandwich at lunch, and a tablespoon of dressing on salad at dinner, you will use three of the recommended fat servings, leaving four for cooking or consumption in prepared food. Vegetables sautéed in oil will carry at least one serving of fat, and a snack bar with 10 grams of fat carries the equivalent of two fat servings. You will see that fat can add up quickly, but it can also be enjoyed just like any other food group.

Free Foods

These are foods that are so low in calories they do not need to be considered in your total food intake. In most cases they do not supply much nutritional value either.

Bouillon, carbonated water and club soda with fruit flavors, coffee, tea, nonstick pan spray, whipped topping (2 tbsp.), horseradish, mustard, pickles, taco sauce, vinegar.

Vegetables (raw 1 c.): cabbage, celery, chinese cabbage, cucumbers, green onions, hot peppers, mushrooms, radishes, zucchini, salad greens including: endive, escarole, lettuce, romaine, spinach.

Seasonings: basil (fresh), celery seeds, chili powder, chives, cinnamon, curry, dill, flavoring extracts (almond, butter, lemon, peppermint, vanilla, walnut), garlic, garlic powder, herbs, hot pepper sauce, lemon, lemon juice, lemon pepper, lime, lime juice, mint, onion powder, oregano, paprika, pepper, pimento, soysauce, spices, wine used in cooking (1/4 cup), Worcestershire sauce.

Combination List

Much of the food we eat is prepared in combination with other ingredients. Here are some simple guidelines to help you determine the food groups carried in mixed dishes.

RECIPE	FOOD GROUP
Casserole, made with noodles, rice, or potato, 1 cup	1 serving bread/starch ½ serving protein-rich
Pizza, cheese, 1 sl.	1 serving bread/starch ½ protein-rich
Macaroni and cheese, 1 cup	2 bread/starch ½ calcium-rich
Fried Food, 3 oz. fish or chicken	1 protein-rich 1 bread/starch 1 fat
Lasagna, cheese, 10 oz. (3-inch square)	2 bread/starch 1 protein-rich 1 vegetable 1 fat
Hamburger, 3 oz. with roll	1 protein-rich 2 bread/starch
Soup, broth-based with noodles or rice, 1 cup	1 bread/starch
Soup, broth-based with vegetables, 1 cup	1 vegetable

Should I Buy Diet Foods?

I have been a dietitian for more than 20 years. In that time Americans have dramatically increased their intake of "diet" foods—and we are fatter today than ever before. Based on my observations, "diet" foods do not help with weight loss, they actually appear to have accomplished the opposite. I recommend that you eat foods that are as close as possible to the way Mother Nature created them. Not only do foods with minimal processing carry more nutrition, they provide more satisfaction. One of the most important keys to good health, whether you are pregnant or not, is the inclusion and enjoyment of good wholesome food in your diet. I would rather see you savor a delicious piece of cheesecake once in a while than repeatedly snack on a heavily processed, refined, no-fat cheesecake lookalike. In the long run, eating the real thing and being thoughtful about it seems to help people lose weight and keep it off.

Daily Option, or Foods That Don't Fit List

The foods listed here provide calories but very little, if any, nutrition. One serving daily provides about 50 calories. The sugar-free alternatives can be used, but since I don't encourage the use of artificial sweeteners (unless you are diabetic), I'd rather see you enjoy the real thing.

maple syrup

jam/jelly

Life Savers

breath mints

regular soda (6 oz.)

sugar, white or brown (1 tbsp.)

honey (1 tbsp.)

chocolate candy (½ oz.)

chocolate syrup (1 tbsp.)

Restaurant Reality

If you eat at restaurants or buy takeout or deli foods more than once a week, you should think carefully before you order. Portion sizes can be significantly higher than when cooking at home. To make eating out more healthful try the following: Choose basic sandwiches. Avoid the "deluxe" and "super" items. Avoid fried foods or those with cream or cheese sauces. Order fruit and vegetables or bring them from home for snacking. Choose bagels, English muffins, or toast rather than donuts and pastry. Many of the restaurant chains have nutritional information available. Ask for it!

Homemade	Restaurant
Muffin, 1 oz., 120 calories	Muffin, 4 oz., 430 calories
Sandwich, 350 calories	Sandwich, 700 calories
Broiled steak, 3 oz. 170 calories	Steak, 16 oz., 900 calories
Pasta, 1 cup with ½ cup tomato sauce, 250 calories	Pasta, 3½ cups, spaghetti with tomato sauce 850 calories

DON'T JUST ASSUME YOU ARE EATING WELL— PROVE IT!

Even if you are gaining weight at a rate that pleases you, I strongly urge all pregnant women to keep a food diary. Spend a few minutes recording what you have eaten in the past 24 hours. Use the form below and put the foods into the categories they belong in. Rare is the person who eats exactly the right number of servings from every food group all the time. You should be looking for patterns in your diet. For example, are you eating the recommended vegetables, fruits and proteins? Are you getting adequate calcium by eating the recommended dairy and calcium sources? Are there a large number of beverages or snacks that carry calories but offer little in the way of nutrition? You really can't answer these questions unless you keep an objective record of what you eat. Evaluate it and strive to add the food your body needs and cut back on the foods you might be overeating. Some women keep food records every day, but most only write down what they eat occasionally, when they feel the need to "spot check." The goal is to balance your menu over a seven-day period.

FOOD DIARY

Time	Food	Amount
Breakfast		
Morning snack		
Lunch		
Afternoon snack		
Dinner		
Evening snack		

Number of food group servings consumed:

Milk _____   Vegetable _____

Meat _____   Starch _____

Fruit _____   Fat _____

Other _____

4

So What Should I Cook?

Good food is essential to good health, during pregnancy as well as after. I define good food as anything that is "real," meaning it has been minimally processed and made from ingredients produced by Mother Nature. In most cases I like to see women, and their families, eating real fruit instead of fruit roll-ups, blueberry muffins made with real blueberries instead of blueberry-flavored Pop-Tarts, or real orange juice instead of powdered orange drink—even if the powder is fortified with vitamins. This preference for real food comes from my belief (and science backs it up) that food carries vital ingredients that go beyond just vitamins, minerals, and protein. When we stray too far from food in its natural state, or rely on manufactured food too often, I fear we may not get optimal nutrition. I also believe real food is more satisfying because it carries fiber and a natural balance of elements that don't promote overeating. Many processed foods carry a dose of sodium or sugar that would never occur naturally, but are added to promote flavor and over-consumption.

The recipes in this section are designed to be easy to prepare and rich in the nutrients pregnant women need, such as vitamins B_6, D, E, folate, iron, calcium, zinc, and magnesium. Most women in the United States obtain a sufficient amount of protein, but their intake of fruits, vegetables, and dairy products is often low. Whenever possible I try to incorporate fruits and vegetables into recipes. Nonfat and low-fat dairy products are specified because the fat has been removed without losing the beneficial calcium it carries. However, women who aren't gaining enough, young women, and women carrying twins may actually need the calories that 2-percent and whole-milk dairy foods can carry. If this is the case, switch to the higher fat dairy foods and there will be no noticeable difference in the final result.

You will also notice that the recipes call for butter instead of margarine. In all cases I keep the amounts of butter low, but I like the taste of butter, and new research suggests that when used in small amounts it is no better or worse for us than equal amounts of margarine.

After each recipe you'll find information about serving size and food groups, which are estimations. When ingredients are used in small amounts (less than an eighth of a portion in the food list), I omit it from the totals. In some cases fat may appear in the food group total per serving even when not included in the ingredient lists. This occurs when ingredients are used in combination and contribute a total of 5 grams of fat to a serving. You'll notice this when cheese (which can carry 7 to 10 grams of fat per ounce) is used as a protein source instead of a lower fat choice like boneless chicken (chicken may carry only 3 to 5 grams of fat per ounce). Remember that the food groupings are to be used only as guidelines, not absolute measurements. Eat when you are hungry, and enjoy what you eat. Use the food groups to guide you when you feel uncertain about your food choices, but don't be a slave to it. These are theoretical recommendations and you may need to eat more food on some days, less on others—listen to your body.

SNACKS

Almost all pregnant women require snacks between meals to keep their energy up. Fruit and yogurt, or fruit and cheese, or milk and a whole-grain cereal or muffin are good choices because they supply the food groups women are often low in. The occasional cookie can satisfy an appetite, too. Watch out for high-fat ice creams, brownies, or chips. Yes, they satisfy an appetite, but they carry a lot of calories and not a whole lot of nutrition. Try some of the snack choices suggested under the Ready-to-Eat list on page 92.

Yogurt and Veggie Dip

⑨

Yogurt is a much better source of calcium than sour cream, making this a delicious and nutritious dip for mothers-to-be.

½ cup nonfat plain yogurt
½ cup non- or low-fat creamy Italian salad dressing
1–2 cups prepared vegetables: peeled carrots, sliced peppers, broccoli florets

1) Combine the yogurt and the dressing and pour into a small bowl.

2) Surround the bowl with the vegetables and serve.

Makes two portions: ¼ calcium, and 1 vegetable per serving.

Curry Topping

🌀

Here is a pleasant way to get your calcium and turn ho-hum vegetables into something more exciting!

    1 cup nonfat yogurt
    1 tbsp. prepared curry powder
    1 tsp. honey
    1 tbsp. raisins

1) In a glass bowl combine all the ingredients, cover and refrigerate for at least 15 minutes or overnight to combine the flavors.

2) Use ¼ cup to top any steamed vegetable such as carrots, broccoli, green beans, or a baked sweet potato.

Makes four ¼ cup portions: ¼ cup calcium per serving.

Roasted Garlic Cheese Topping or Dip

🌀

When garlic is roasted it is no longer pungent but mild without being dull. Combined with ricotta this makes a much better calcium source than traditional sour cream– or cream cheese–based dips. Use this as a dip with vegetables, or even tossed with hot pasta.

    1 garlic bulb (the entire head)
    1 cup ricotta cheese
    1 tbsp. milk or cream for thinning (optional)

1) Preheat the oven to 350°F. Wrap the garlic in aluminum foil and bake for one hour. Allow it to cool.

2) Remove from the foil and pinch each clove so the garlic slips out into a clean glass bowl.

3) Stir in the ricotta cheese and blend well. Serve right away on top of a baked potato, or refrigerate, covered until ready to use. If using as a dip or a pasta topping, thin the cheese mixture with the milk or cream. This tastes best when served warm.

Makes 1 cup: 1 calcium serving per recipe.

Sweet Potato Chips

⛎

Here is an alternative to french fries and potato chips that carries more nutrition because it is made with sweet potatoes and baked, not fried.

   2 sweet potatoes

1) Preheat oven to 375°F. Peel the potatoes and slice ⅛ inch thick.

2) Arrange in a single layer on a cookie sheet and spray lightly with vegetable oil. Flip the potatoes and lightly spray the other side.

3) Bake for 15 to 18 minutes or until crisp, turning once, halfway through the cooking time. Salt to taste, and serve plain or with a prepared or homemade salsa.

Makes two large portions: 2 vegetables per serving.

Salsa

Make this in the summer months when tomatoes are inexpensive and oh so good! During the winter use bottled salsa. All salsa is low in fat and rich in vitamin C. Try salsa with baked tortillas or crackers instead of the traditional fried chips.

    4 whole tomatoes, washed and chopped
    3 scallions, trimmed and chopped
    1 tbsp. vegetable oil
    ¼ cup corriander, leaves chopped coarsely
    5 olives, black or green, minced
    Lemon juice to taste

1) Combine all the ingredients in a glass bowl. Cover and refrigerate for at least one hour before serving.

Makes two cups: 1 vegetable per ½ cup serving.

Ready-to-Eat Snacks that Are Good for Mom and Baby

Graham crackers	Fresh fruit
Whole-wheat crackers	Rice Cakes
Pretzels	Whole-grain cereal
Canned fruit packed in juice	Bagels
Low-fat chocolate milk	Dried fruit: raisins, apples, apricots
Fruited yogurt	String cheese
Whole-wheat toast with peanut butter	Whole-grain cereal with fruit and milk
Applesauce	Peanuts or almonds (¼ c.)
Homemade muffins	Carrot sticks

SOUP

Serve soup with a glass of milk, a slice of bread, fruit for dessert, and you have a complete dinner. Homemade versions are often more nutritious because you can control the quality and quantity of ingredients. Store-bought brands can be high in fat and sodium, and skimp on nutritious ingredients like protein and fresh vegetables.

Don't Forget Sandwiches

People are always asking for advice on how to serve healthy food when they are in a hurry or on the run.

Sandwiches are one of my favorite solutions. Start with a roll or sliced bread (preferably whole wheat). Then fill it with a generous serving of crisp vegetables, such as the familiar lettuce and tomato, or the less traditional, such as thinly sliced carrots, cucumbers, peppers, red or white onions, even finely chopped broccoli or zucchini. Use whatever vegetable combination you like. Add a protein source, which can be a slice of cheese, chicken, turkey, or lean beef, even sliced tofu, a nut butter, or tahini. For flavor add a zesty mustard or a bit of mayonnaise or salad dressing and enjoy!

Chicken Barley Soup

◉

Barley is a good source of protein and fiber that cooks into a tender, soft grain. Serve this soup with some crusty bread and a glass of milk or sliced cheese, and with fruit for dessert, you have a perfectly balanced meal.

1 small onion
4 cups prepared chicken broth
¾ cup pearled barley
2 carrots, grated
1 cup sliced mushrooms
1 cup cooked chicken, chopped

1) In a soup pot, bring ¼ cup of the broth to a boil and sauté the onions for three minutes on medium heat

until tender and translucent. Pour in the remaining broth and add the barley, carrots, and mushrooms. Cover and simmer on medium heat for 30 minutes. Stir occasionally.

2) Taste the barley. When it is soft and tender, stir in the chicken and cook on low for five minutes until thoroughly heated through. Serve warm.

Makes 4 cups of soup equal to: 1 bread/starch, 1 vegetable, and ½ protein per serving.

Very Vegetable Soup

◎

This is a recipe for mothers who don't often eat all the veggies they should. It makes use of an assortment of vegetables. Serve it with a good protein source such as a glass of milk, a slice of hearty bread with peanut butter, or grate an ounce or two of sharp cheese over your bowl before serving.

1 onion, chopped
2 cloves of garlic, chopped
1 tbsp. vegetable oil
1 cup carrots, peeled and chopped
2 red potatoes, chopped into 2-inch cubes
1 cup green beans, chopped
1 cup corn niblets
1 13-ounce can of tomatoes, chopped
4 cups of prepared chicken broth
6 whole peppercorns

1) In a large saucepan, sauté the onions and the garlic in the oil until soft and translucent, about three minutes.

2) Stir in all remaining ingredients and simmer, covered, for 30 minutes until potatoes are tender when pierced with a fork. Serve warm.

Makes 6 1-cup portions: 2 vegetables per serving.

Spinach Soup

Here is another way to get those green leafy vegetables that are so good for pregnant women.

1 small onion
2 tsp. vegetable oil
1 pound fresh spinach, rinsed and trimmed of dry hard stems
3 cups homemade or prepared chicken broth
1 cup cooked orzo noodles

1) In a heavy soup pot or Dutch oven sauté the onion in the oil until it is soft but not brown.

2) Add the spinach and the broth. Cover and cook on low-medium heat for 15 minutes.

3) Stir in the cooked orzo and cook for five minutes more, until the orzo is heated through. Serve hot.

Makes four portions: 1 bread/starch and 1 vegetable per serving.

Fish Chowder

✆

The advantages of this recipe abound. This is a great way to prepare fish in a tasty and wholesome manner. Plus the milk used is extra calcium, which is a great bonus.

> 1 pound white fish such as haddock, halibut, or cod, fresh or frozen
> 2 tbsp. butter
> 1 medium onion, sliced
> 4 new potatoes, quartered
> 2 cups water
> 2 cups evaporated milk (preferably skim)
> Salt and pepper to taste
> 3 tbsp. flour (optional)

1) Chop the fish into cubes and set aside.

2) In a two-quart soup pot melt the butter, add the onion, and cook for two minutes until soft.

3) Add the water and potatoes, bring to a boil, cook for five minutes.

4) Add the fish and milk, stir, cover, and cook for 20 minutes on low to medium heat. Do not boil.

5) Add salt and pepper to taste. Serve warm. For a thicker chowder sift the flour over the mixture, stir and cook for three to five minutes.

Makes four portions: 1 protein, 1 calcium, 1 bread/starch and 1 fat per serving.

Lentil Sausage Soup

◎

Lentils, which are somewhat bland in flavor, benefit when combined with a spicier food like Italian sausage.

    2 cups uncooked lentils
    1 tbsp. vegetable oil
    8 oz. sweet Italian sausage, chopped
    1 onion, chopped
    2 carrots, peeled and chopped coarsely
    1 12-ounce can chicken broth
    1 bay leaf

1) Soak the lentils in water overnight and rinse thoroughly, or boil in 6–8 cups water for 30–40 minutes, drain and rinse.

2) In a heavy soup pot sauté the sausage and onion in the oil for five minutes until it is no longer pink. Drain fat.

3) Add the carrots, rinsed lentils, broth, bay leaf, and enough water to cover the ingredients by 1 inch.

4) Bring to a boil. Simmer, covered, on low heat for 45 minutes. Serve hot.

Makes 4 portions: 1 protein, 1 vegetable, 1 fat per serving.

Great Greens

🌀

Pregnant women are advised to eat lots of green leafy vegetables, which contain generous amounts of folic acid, iron, and calcium. Spinach can carry a large amount of naturally occurring oxalic acid, believed to block calcium absorption, but it's still a good source of iron and fiber. Use greens in a salad or try this versatile cooking method. It works with all sorts of green leafy vegetables.

> 1 pound spinach, kale, collards, or beet greens
> 1 tbsp. olive oil
> 2–4 cloves garlic, chopped
> 2 tbsp. water
> Salt
> Pepper
> 2–4 tbsp. cider vinegar (optional)

1) Wash the greens thoroughly. (They are almost always gritty and require several washings.) Remove the thick, coarse stems and any dry or discolored leaves. Chop coarsely.

2) In a large skillet sauté the garlic in the oil for one minute. Add the prepared greens and the water. Cover and let simmer for four minutes. Season with salt and pepper. Serve warm, with a drizzle of vinegar if desired.

Makes two portions: 1 vegetable per serving.

Spinach Mornay

🌀

Baked vegetables are so satisfying, particularly in cold weather. Serve this as a side dish with any cooked meat or poultry dish.

1 pound fresh spinach washed and hard stems removed
1 tbsp. butter
2 tbsp. all purpose flour
1 cup low-fat milk
½ cup cheddar cheese, grated

1) Preheat oven to 350°F. Blanch the spinach in boiling water for two minutes. Drain and rinse with cold water and set aside.

2) In a saucepan melt the butter, stir in the flour, and cook on medium heat for two minutes. Slowly add the milk, stirring to blend ingredients. Cook for 8–10 minutes until the mixture starts to thicken. Do not let it boil and don't let it burn. Stir in the cheese and remove from the heat.

3) Place the spinach in a lightly oiled casserole dish. Pour the mornay sauce over the spinach and bake until the sauce bubbles and is lightly browned, about 20 minutes.

Makes two large portions: 2 vegetable, ½ calcium, ½ protein, and 2 fat per serving.

Glorious Greens

✆

Preparing collards, beet greens, or spinach in the microwave oven is fast and tasty.

1 pound fresh greens, washed and drained, trim off tough stems
2 tbsp. water or chicken broth

1) Place greens along with the liquid in a one-quart microwave-safe dish. Cover and cook on full power for two minutes. Stir and let stand for two minutes, covered before serving. Serve hot, topped with a sprinkle of lemon, balsamic vinegar, or a tablespoon of your favorite grated cheese.

Makes four portions: 1 vegetable per serving.

GREAT GRAINS

Grains are a delicious, low-fat way to get the fiber you need along with important nutrients including magnesium, B vitamins, folic acid, zinc, and copper. A diet that incorporates grains every day can reduce the risk of cancer and heart disease. While pregnant, you want to eat at least seven to eight servings of grain or starchy foods daily, but strive for a total of 11 servings and make three of those whole grains. Whole grains are grains that have not had their outer shell removed, and their bran coating carries lots of nutrition. Three servings might sound like a lot, but two slices of whole-wheat bread in a sandwich and half a cup of brown rice or cooked oatmeal is all it takes to meet that three-servings-a-day recommendation.

Whole-Grain and Bean Tip

For good health, pregnant or not, adults should eat three whole-grain foods daily and beans at least once per week. To make this easier, keep a supply of canned beans and instant brown rice in the cupboard. Try the following combination: Mix together 1 cup cooked brown rice, 1 16-ounce can of drained and rinsed beans (black beans and black-eyed peas are my favorite), 1 16-ounce can drained unsalted corn, and ½ cup prepared salsa. Mix together and serve cold or bake in the oven until hot and top with grated cheese. This combination is packed with nutrition and can be ready in seconds.

Barley Risotto
🌀

Barley is a grain rich in fiber and protein. I assemble this dish, get it started and tend to it while I organize dinner.

1 tsp. butter
1 whole onion, peeled and chopped
1 cup broccoli, chopped
1 cup carrots, peeled and chopped
4 cups homemade or canned chicken broth
1½ cup pearl barley

Pepper to taste
4 ounces cheddar cheese, grated

1) In a large sauté pan melt the butter, add the onion, and cook for one minute.

2) Add the broccoli and carrots. Sauté until just tender, about four minutes, then remove vegetables from the pan and set aside.

3) In the same pan add the barley along with ¼ cup of the broth and sauté for two minutes.

4) Add enough additional broth (about 1 cup) to just cover the barley, stir and let simmer uncovered on medium heat. When the broth is absorbed (about three minutes), add another half cup of broth, stir and simmer until the liquid is absorbed again. Continue this process until all the broth has been added. If the barley is not cooked, add additional liquid (about ½ cup of water or broth). Do not let the barley burn or dry out. Once the liquid is absorbed the barley should be plump and tender. Add the cooked vegetables, and cover for five minutes to reheat.

5) Add pepper to taste and sprinkle with the cheese before serving. Serve hot.

Makes two large portions: 3 bread/starch, 1 protein, 2 vegetable, and 2 fats per serving.

Whole-grain Pilaf

⊚

Most of us do not eat the three servings of whole-grain foods that nutrition experts advise. This is a recipe that can be used with brown rice, pearl barley, or a combination of these grains. It is a tasty way to eat whole grains. (Note: With grains, age affects cooking time, so the older the grain the longer it will need to cook.)

½ cup onion, chopped
1 clove garlic, chopped
1 tbsp. olive oil
1 cup pearl barley or brown rice
2 cups prepared chicken broth
1 fresh lemon for garnish
1 10-ounce package of frozen chopped spinach, thawed, or 1 cup frozen peas, thawed

1) Sauté the onion and garlic in the oil until softened.

2) Stir in the grain and sauté another minute or two.

3) Stir in the broth and bring it to a boil, then reduce heat and cover. Cook on low heat for 45 minutes.

4) Test the mixture. If the grains look dry, add ½ cup water. The grains should be soft and tender but not mushy.

5) Stir in the vegetables, cover, and cook another five minutes or until the vegetables are heated through.

Makes four portions: 1 bread/starch and 1 vegetable per serving.

Wheat Berry–Rice Combo

⑨

Few people include wheat berries as a cooking staple. I serve this because I like the unusual taste and texture of this combination. It's good for us, too!

½ cup whole-wheat berries
½ cup brown rice
1 tsp. butter
2 cups water
Salt to taste

1) Bring the water to a boil. Add the butter. Slowly pour in the rice and wheat berries at a rate that allows the water to keep boiling (this helps prevent clumping). Stir once, cover, and reduce heat to low. Cook for 35 minutes, then check the mixture. Both the wheat berries and the brown rice should be soft and tender. If they are not, cook an additional five to ten minutes, adding more liquid to prevent scorching. Fluff with a fork before serving.

Makes four portions: 1 bread/starch per serving.

Quinoa (pronounced "keenwa")

⑥

This is an unrefined grain originally cultivated in South Africa and now available in health-food stores and specialty shops. A ½ cup uncooked portion carries over 7 grams of dietary fiber and a generous dose of magnesium. Serve it instead of rice.

> ½ cup quinoa
> 1 cup water
> 1 tsp. butter
> Salt and pepper to taste

1) In a skillet, toast the uncooked grain on medium heat for three to four minutes until it darkens slightly in color. Remove from heat and set aside.

2) In a medium saucepan with a cover, bring the water and the butter to a boil. Add the toasted quinoa, return to a boil, stir once, and cook covered for 20 minutes, until tender. Fluff with a fork and serve with salt and pepper to taste.

Makes two half-cup portions: 1 bread/starch per serving.

MEATLESS ENTREES

A meal does not need to include meat to provide protein. Pasta and grain foods carry about 2 grams of protein for each half-cup portion. When combined with egg, cheese, or milk they become a very good source of protein.

Tofu Tip

Tofu is being credited with preventing heart disease, relieving menopause symptoms, and providing calcium and protein. The easiest way I know to serve tofu is to cut it into small cubes, pour chicken broth over it, and warm it in the microwave. Sprinkle with soy sauce and chopped scallions and enjoy!

Vegetarian Meatloaf

🌀

Cooked barley forms the foundation of this main dish meal. Serve it with ketchup as with traditional meatloaf or try a salsa or Italian tomato sauce.

½ cup pearl barley
1 tbsp. butter
1 small onion, chopped
½ pound mushrooms, chopped
3 carrots, peeled and shredded
4 oz. cheddar cheese shredded
2 large eggs, beaten
½ tsp. dried thyme
½ tsp. oregano
Salt and pepper

1) Cook the barley in 2 cups boiling salted water until tender, about 30 to 40 minutes, drain and set aside.

2)   Preheat the oven to 350°F. Lightly oil an 8" x 4" loaf
pan.

3)   In a large skillet sauté the vegetables in the butter for 8
to 10 minutes, until tender. Remove from heat, add the
barley, seasonings, salt and pepper to taste.

4)   Mix the eggs and cheese into the barley mixture until
well blended and pour into the prepared loaf pan. Bake
for 60 minutes until firm and lightly browned on top.
Slice and serve hot with ketchup, cheese sauce, salsa or
tomato sauce.

*Makes four portions: 1 protein, 1 bread/starch, 1 vegetable,
and 1 fat per serving.*

Easy Spinach Tortillas
⑨

Another meatless meal that gets protein from the combination of cheeses and a healthy dose of calcium, too.

6 soft flour tortillas
1 pound frozen chopped spinach, thawed and
drained
1 egg
1 cup low-fat cottage cheese
½ cup cheddar cheese, grated
Fresh ground black pepper

1) Preheat the oven to 350°F. In a glass bowl combine the spinach, cottage and cheddar cheeses, pepper and eggs until well blended.

2) Place an equal amount of the spinach mixture in each tortilla, fold and place on a cookie sheet. Cover with foil and bake for 20 minutes until hot and the cheese is melted.

Makes six portions: 1 bread/starch, 1 calcium, and 1 vegetable per serving.

Baked Couscous with Sautéed Vegetables

◎

Couscous is sold in bulk containers at the health-food store and in prepackaged boxes. There are refined and whole-grain varieties. I recommend the whole grain because it carries more nutrition, but both are delicious and easy to prepare.

1 12-oz. package of couscous
1 tbsp. vegetable oil
1 clove garlic, minced
1 medium onion, sliced
1 green pepper, seeded and sliced
1 cup mushrooms, sliced
1 small bunch broccoli, chopped
1 carrot, peeled and sliced
½ cup fresh basil, chopped
8 oz. Monterey Jack cheese, grated
¼ cup chicken or vegetable broth

1) Preheat the oven to 350°F. Prepare the couscous as directed on the package. When cooked, spread onto a lightly oiled lasagne dish and set aside.

2) In a large skillet sauté the onion and garlic in the oil for one minute. Add the remaining vegetables and basil, cook on low heat until tender but not mushy, about five minutes. To speed cooking cover the skillet, but don't overcook.

3) Spread the vegetables and broth over the couscous and sprinkle with the cheese. Cover with aluminum foil and bake for ten to fifteen minutes until hot and cheese melts. Serve while hot.

Makes 6 portions: 2 bread/starch, 1½ vegetable, 1 calcium.

Main Dish Potatoes

🌀

I think of this as a quick hot lunch when eating alone, but it can be served as a main dish at supper. Just multiply the ingredients by the number of guests at the table.

1 large potato
4 oz. of your favorite low-fat cheese such as mozzarella or cheddar, grated
2 tbsp. low-fat milk
½ cup cooked broccoli, chopped

1) Prick the potato with a fork. Cook in the microwave for four minutes. It should feel soft when done. Let rest until cool enough to handle.

2) Slice in half and scoop out the potato without tearing the skin. Combine the cooked potato with all other ingredients until well blended.

3) Fill the potato skins with the potato, broccoli and cheese mixture. Bake at 350°F on a baking sheet until top is browned, about ten minutes. Serve hot.

Makes one portion: 1 bread/starch, 1 protein, 1 vegetable and 1 fat per serving.

PASTA

Pasta can be the foundation of a very healthy meal. Experiment with a variety of toppings. For convenience try the store-bought products such as pesto sauce and white clam sauce. Even the cans of prepared tomatoes can be tossed with fresh-cooked pasta to form a simple, but fast and healthy, meal.

Garbanzo Bean and Broccoli Rabe Pasta

☞

This is a wonderful meatless main dish. It contains nutrients that new mothers really need, like folic acid, protein, and fiber.

1 pound broccoli rabe
1 tbsp. olive oil
2 garlic cloves, chopped
1 15-oz. can garbanzo beans, drained and rinsed
8 oz. Rotini pasta noodles
Salt and pepper to taste
Fresh grated parmesan to taste

1)   Wash the broccoli rabe and chop it coarsely. Bring two
     quarts of water to a boil. Plunge the broccoli rabe into
     the water and cook for four minutes. Drain and rinse
     with cold water, set aside.

2)   In a skillet sauté the garlic in the oil for three minutes,
     until lightly browned. Add the broccoli rabe, toss with
     the oil and add the garbanzo beans. Cover and turn the
     heat to low.

3)   Cook the pasta as directed on the package. Drain and
     toss with the cooked broccoli rabe/bean mixture. Add
     salt and pepper to taste. Serve hot with grated cheese.

*Makes two portions: 1 protein, 2 vegetable and 4
bread/starch per serving.*

Summer Pasta

This is best in summer when tomatoes can be picked from
the garden and fresh basil is in abundance. The fresh mozzarella cheese provides a good source of protein and calories.
The tomatoes are a delicious way to get vitamin C.

1 pound fresh tomatoes, washed, chopped, and
lightly salted
1 cup fresh basil leaves, rinsed and chopped
2 tbsp. olive oil
1 clove garlic, finely minced
8 oz. spaghetti
1 pound fresh mozzarella cheese, chopped into ½-
inch cubes
Salt and pepper
10 Greek olives, pitted and chopped

1) Combine the tomatoes, basil, garlic, and oil. Toss together and set aside.

2) Cook the pasta according to package instructions, rinse
and pour into a pasta bowl. Add tomato mixture, toss,
season with salt and pepper if desired. Sprinkle with the
mozzarella cheese and olives before serving. Serve immediately.

*Makes four portions: 2 bread/starch, 1 vegetable, 1 fat, and
½ protein per serving.*

Baked Macaroni and Cheese
◎

This dish is almost as easy as the prepackaged type, but the
addition of cottage cheese makes it richer in protein and
calcium.

8 ounces elbow macaroni
2 tbsp. butter
3 tbsp. all-purpose flour
2 cups low-fat milk
1 tbsp. prepared mustard
½ cup grated Parmesan cheese
1 cup low-fat cottage cheese

1) Cook the pasta as described on the package. Drain, rinse, and set aside.

2) In a medium saucepan melt the butter, stir in the flour, and cook for one minute. Slowly add the milk and stir until it starts to thicken, about five minutes. Stir in the cheese and stir until well blended.

3) Pour the cooked pasta into a small, lightly buttered casserole dish. Pour the milk/cheese mixture over the pasta and stir well. Place in the oven and bake for 20 minutes until golden and bubbly.

Makes four portions: 2 bread/starch, ½ calcium, ½ protein, 1½ fat per serving.

Pasta with Tomato Meat Sauce
◎

Spaghetti and tomato sauce is still one of the easiest meals to assemble and a good food to eat while pregnant. It carries lots of carbohydrates for energy, iron for you and the baby, and vitamin C, which helps your body absorb the iron better.

1 tbsp. olive oil
1 small onion
2 cloves garlic, minced
8 oz. lean ground beef
1 28-ounce can peeled, crushed tomatoes
8 oz. spaghetti

1) In a large skillet cook the onion and garlic in the oil until
   it softens, about two to three minutes. Add the ground
   beef and cook until it is no longer pink. Drain the fat and
   add the tomatoes. Cover and simmer for 20 minutes.

2) Prepare the spaghetti as directed on the package. Drain
   and pour the meat sauce over the pasta. Serve hot.

*Makes four portions: 2 bread/starch, 1 protein, 2 vegeta-
bles, and 1 fat per serving.*

Spaghetti with Vegetable Sauce

⑨

For a healthy change of taste, try this sauce as an alternative to tomato sauce.

8 oz. spaghetti
1 tbsp. olive oil
1 small onion, chopped
2 cloves garlic, chopped
1 pound spinach or broccoli, washed and trimmed or
frozen and thawed
1 cup chicken broth
¼ cup Parmesan cheese
Salt and pepper to taste

1) In a large skillet sauté the onion and the garlic for two minutes. Add the spinach or broccoli (or a combination) and cook until soft and tender, about 5–7 minutes.

2) Pour the cooked vegetable into a food processor and puree, adding enough broth to make a smooth sauce.

3) Prepare the spaghetti as directed on the package. Drain and top with the vegetable sauce and grated cheese. Serve while hot.

Makes four portions: 2 bread/starch, 1 vegetable, 1 fat per serving.

FISH

Seafood is a delicious source of protein and almost always contains less fat than beef or chicken. Fresh fish should carry a pleasant ocean smell. Frozen fish is often more economical and equally nutritious. Try to eat fish at least once per week for the health benefits it can provide.

Shrimp Scampi with Vegetables

◎

The traditional scampi made with gobs of butter is too rich to have on a regular basis. This recipe still calls for garlic and some butter, but vegetables are added to boost flavor and nutrition.

1 tbsp. butter
3 cloves garlic, chopped
2 carrots, peeled and sliced into slivers
½ pound chinese pea pods, stems removed
1 pound shrimp, deveined and cleaned
2 tbsp. prepared chicken broth or water
10 whole cherry tomatoes
Fresh grated Parmesan cheese
12 oz. fettucine noodles, cooked

1) In a large skillet sauté the garlic in the butter for two minutes. Add the carrots and pea pods and cook for two minutes more.

2) Add the shrimp and broth or water to the vegetables and cook until white and firm, about 5–6 minutes. Just before serving, stir in the whole tomatoes, cover and let sit for one minute before pouring over prepared pasta. Serve with the grated cheese.

Makes four portions: 1 protein, 3 bread/starch, 2 vegetables, and 1 fat per serving.

Crusty Salmon Fillet

⑨

Prepared as directed in this recipe your fish will come out moist and tender. If you like the taste of horseradish (as I do), double or even triple the amount called for.

1 pound salmon fillet with skin
1 tbsp. mayonnaise

½ tbsp. prepared horseradish
⅓ cup seasoned bread crumbs
1 tsp. lemon peel, grated

1) Preheat the oven to 350°F. Place the fillet on a baking sheet, skin side down.

2) In a glass bowl combine all remaining ingredients until well blended. With a spoon or clean fingers pat the mixture over the fish so the entire fillet is covered.

3) Bake for 10–12 minutes, until the fish flakes and it is firm to the touch.

Makes four portions: 1 protein per serving.

Tuna Pot Pie
🌀

Almost every cupboard in America carries a can or two of tuna. Use this recipe when you want to put together a warm satisfying meal in a hurry.

1 tbsp. butter
1 small onion, finely chopped
1 cup celery, chopped
4 tsp. all-purpose flour
1 cup prepared chicken broth
½ cup milk
½ cup peas, fresh or frozen
½ cup corn, fresh or frozen

¼ cup cheddar cheese, grated
2 6.5-ounce cans water-packed tuna, drained

Topping:
4 slices bread, white or whole wheat
¼ cup milk
1 egg, beaten
1 tbsp. cheddar cheese, grated

1) Preheat oven to 375°F. In a large skillet cook the onion and celery in the butter until soft.

2) Stir in the flour and cook for one minute. Add the broth and the milk and cook for five minutes. The mixture will start to thicken.

3) Add the cheese, corn, and peas. Fold in the tuna.

4) Pour the tuna mixture into a lightly oiled casserole dish.

5) *For the topping* beat together the egg and milk. Dip the bread into the milk mixture, then place on top of the tuna mixture. Do this with each slice until all the top is covered, overlapping or cutting the bread as needed. Sprinkle with cheese.

6) Bake uncovered for 25 minutes, until the mixture is completely cooked and the bread is lightly browned.

Makes four portions: 4 bread/starch, 1 fat, 1 vegetable, ¼ calcium, and 1 protein per serving.

POULTRY

Chicken and turkey are probably the poultry we prepare most often. The white meat is usually leaner than the dark, but the dark meat contains more nutrients, especially iron. Cooks will be happy to know you can cook your poultry with the skin on and remove it after. The fat cooks away from the meat. It does not get "soaked up." All poultry products have the potential to carry dangerous bacteria, so always cook poultry to an internal temperature of 180°F and until juices run clear. Do not let any uncooked juices mingle with raw foods and be sure to clean cutting boards and other surfaces thoroughly after handling raw poultry.

Turkey Kabobs

ⓢ

These tender cubes of turkey are packed with protein and they are also a good source of zinc. Serve them over a bed of brown rice or the Wheat Berry–Rice Combo on page 104.

1 8-oz. boneless turkey breast
2 small onions
1 green pepper
6 whole mushrooms
8 cherry tomatoes
1 cup prepared Italian dressing

1) Cut the turkey into eight evenly sized cubes. Peel the onion and slice in half. Seed the pepper and cut into six

equal pieces. Put all the turkey, onion, peppers, mushrooms, and tomatoes in a large glass bowl. Add the dressing and stir gently to coat all the ingredients. Refrigerate for at least one hour, up to three hours.

2)　On ten-inch skewers, alternate the turkey with the fresh vegetables, using an equal amount on each skewer.

3)　Preheat the broiler. Place the kabobs on a baking sheet and broil 15 minutes, turning at least once. Turkey should be firm when cooked and vegetables lightly browned.

Makes two portions: 1 protein, 2 vegetables, and 1 fat per serving.

Baked Marinated Chicken with Vegetables

◎

I try to make cooking efficient whenever I can. This dish cooks chicken along with potatoes and carrots, making a complete one-dish meal.

　　1 3½-pound chicken, cut up, skin removed
　　1 cup prepared Italian dressing
　　4 baking potatoes
　　4 large carrots, peeled and cut in half
　　2 tbsp. all-purpose flour
　　1 chicken bouillon cube
　　1 cup water

1) Rinse the chicken and place it in a glass bowl. Pour the dressing on top, stir to coat all pieces. Refrigerate and marinate for 1–3 hours.

2) Preheat oven to 350°F. Arrange the chicken in a roasting pan along with the potatoes and carrots. Bake 40–45 minutes, until chicken is cooked and juices run clear.

3) Remove the chicken and cooked vegetables to a heated platter. Drain as much surface grease from the roasting pan as you can. Stir the flour into the pan drippings. Add the water and bouillon cube, and stir over low heat until the gravy is thick. Serve with the chicken.

Makes four portions: 1 protein, 1 vegetable, 2 bread/starch, and 1 fat per serving.

Chicken Cacciatore

🌀

Batches of this can be prepared and frozen for later use. Just double or triple the ingredients to meet your needs. Serve this over cooked pasta for a terrific meal.

2 whole boneless, skinless chicken breasts, about 1 pound
1 cup prepared Italian bread crumbs
Vegetable or olive oil spray
1 cup sliced mushrooms
1 zucchini, sliced
1 green pepper, chopped

1 jar prepared tomato sauce
1 pound cooked spaghetti or fettucine

1) Preheat the oven to 350°F. Cut the chicken into four even pieces. Rinse and dredge in the bread crumbs. In a large skillet coated with vegetable spray add the chicken and cook until browned on all sides. Transfer to a lightly oiled casserole dish.

2) Add all the prepared vegetables to the skillet and sauté until just softened.

3) Distribute the vegetables over the chicken and pour the tomato sauce over the top, arranging the chicken so all pieces are covered with some of the sauce.

4) Bake for 35–40 minutes or until chicken is cooked. Serve over hot pasta.

Makes four portions: 1 protein, 1 vegetable, 4 bread/starch, and 1 fat per serving.

Steamed Chicken
⑨

This is a dish to rely on when you have no time to cook but crave a home-cooked meal. Once again, it's a complete meal in one pot, making preparation and cleanup very easy.

1 3½-pound broiler chicken, rinsed, gizzards and neck removed
2 cups prepared chicken broth

1 whole onion, peeled
4 large carrots, peeled
4 baking potatoes, cut in half

1) Preheat oven to 350°F. Place the chicken and the onion in a Dutch oven. Pour the broth over the chicken, cover and place in the preheated oven. Bake covered for 30 minutes.

2) Add the vegetables, cover and continue cooking until chicken is cooked and potatoes are tender when pierced with a fork, about 25 minutes more. Serve hot.

Makes 6 portions; 1 protein, 1 bread/starch, 1 vegetable per serving.

Chicken Baked with Lemon

⑨

Chicken is a lean source of protein when it is baked rather than fried. Lemon gives this dish an unexpected but delightful flavor.

1 whole chicken, cut up and rinsed
1 cup prepared chicken broth
1 tsp. or more garlic powder
Fresh pepper
1 lemon, sliced thinly

1) Preheat oven to 350°F. Place the chicken in a flat casserole dish. Sprinkle with the garlic powder. Top with the lemon slices and pour the broth over the chicken.

2) Bake until done, about 45 minutes or until all the juices run clear. Remove lemon before serving.

Makes 6 portions: 1 protein per portion.

BEEF AND PORK

Beef carries impressive amounts of B_{12}, iron, and zinc. Prime and choice cuts carry the most fat. Look for beef marked "select," which is usually the leanest and equal to the higher-fat cuts in protein. Pork is an equally good source of protein and it carries the distinction of being one of the best meat sources of thiamin, one of the B-complex vitamins.

New England Pot Roast

◎

This is a dish that has served new mothers for centuries. It is easy and delicious. Make it ahead and keep it refrigerated so that it is ready for reheating when you get home from a busy day.

    3 pounds beef chuck or rump roast
    ¾ cup all-purpose flour
    Salt and pepper
    1 tbsp. vegetable oil
    1 onion, chopped
    5 large carrots, 1 peeled and chopped, 4 whole
    ½ cup red wine (optional)
    3 cups water
    4 potatoes

1) Preheat oven to 350°F. Put the flour in a clean plastic bag, season with salt and pepper. Add the roast and shake to coat all sides of the meat.

2) In a large Dutch oven or heavy roasting pot, heat the oil and brown the meat on all sides. Add the chopped onion, chopped carrot, water, and wine.

3) Bring to a boil, cover, and transfer to the preheated oven. Cook for three hours. Check the roast every hour, and add more water if needed. Be careful not to let the roast dry out.

4) In the last 40 minutes of cooking, wash the potatoes and carrots and add them to the pot. Cook until the potatoes are tender when pierced with a fork. Serve hot or allow to cool and refrigerate to reheat at a later time.

Each 3-ounce portion: 1 protein, 1 bread/starch (for the potato), and 1 vegetable (for the carrot).

Vegetable Stir Fry with Pork and Tofu

☙

Tofu is being credited with all sorts of health benefits but most American women are unfamiliar with it. When combined with lean meats it extends the protein value of a meal.

1 16-oz. block of firm tofu
8 oz. pork tenderloin or boneless pork chop
1 tbsp. vegetable oil

1 onion, chopped
2 cloves garlic, chopped
1 tbsp. fresh ginger, minced
2 tbsp. soy sauce
2 cups bok choy, sliced, chopped
2 cups fresh broccoli, chopped
1 8-ounce can water chestnuts, sliced
4 cups cooked rice, brown or white

1) Drain the tofu, cut into bite-size cubes, and set aside. Slice the pork into into ¼-inch strips about 2 inches long.

2) In a heavy skillet heat the oil, sauté the onion, garlic, and ginger for three minutes until soft. Add the pork and cook for three minutes on high heat until it is no longer pink. Remove the meat and other ingredients from the pan and set aside. Add the tofu and cook, until browned on all sides about three minutes a side. Remove and set aside. Add the bok choy and broccoli. Cook for three minutes or longer until tender. Return the pork mixture and tofu to the pan and add the soy sauce. Heat through for three minutes. Serve over rice.

Makes four portions: 1 protein, 2 bread/starch, 4 vegetables, 1 fat per serving.

South of the Border Shepherds Pie

◎

Mexican food is becoming America's favorite ethnic food choice, gaining on Italian cuisine. This is an easy and nutritious dish, packed with protein and vegetables.

3 large baking potatoes, peeled and chopped
2 tsp. vegetable oil
1 medium onion, chopped
2 cloves garlic, chopped
2 tsp. ground cumin
1 tbsp. chile powder
1 pound lean ground beef
1 16-oz. can black beans, rinsed and drained
1½ cups frozen corn, thawed
3 tbsp. prepared salsa
½ cup milk
1 tbsp. butter

1) Preheat oven to 350°F. Put the potatoes in a large pot. Add enough water to cover them, along with a sprinkle of salt. Bring to a boil and cook until tender, about 15 minutes.

2) While the potatoes cook. Heat the oil in a large skillet, add the onion and garlic, and cook for one minute. Add the ground beef and sauté until the beef is no longer pink. Drain the fat. Stir in the seasoning, beans and corn. Remove from heat and set aside.

3) When the potatoes are tender, drain and mash with ½ cup milk and 1 tbsp. butter.

4) Lightly oil an oven-proof casserole dish. Pour in the meat mixture and cover with the mashed potatoes. Bake for 20–30 minutes, until the potatoes are just lightly browned.

Makes five portions: 1 protein, 2 bread/starch, 1 fat, and 1 vegetable per serving.

Tortilla Pie

✆

Flour tortillas when cooked in a casserole like this take on the characteristics of a lasagne noodle. Only in this "lasagne" you do not need to precook any pasta.

1 pound lean ground beef
1 15-ounce can kidney beans, drained and rinsed
1 package taco seasoning mix (1.25 oz. net wet)
½ cup water
1 cup prepared salsa or 1 cup chopped fresh tomatoes
1 cup frozen corn, thawed
4–6 soft 6-inch flour tortillas
2 cups low-fat cheddar cheese, shredded

Topping
1 cup lettuce, shredded
½ cup prepared salsa

1) Preheat oven to 350°F. In a medium-size skillet combine the beef, beans, taco seasoning, and water. Sauté,

breaking up any large lumps of ground beef and cook until there are no traces of pink. Drain excess fat.

2) Lightly oil a casserole dish or a lasagne pan. Line the bottom of the dish with two tortillas, cut or tear the tortillas to fit the shape of your pan. Pour in one-third of the meat/bean mixture, ⅓ cup of the corn, ½ cup cheese, and ⅓ cup of the salsa or tomatoes. Repeat this until you have made three layers of tortilla, finishing with the meat, salsa, corn, and cheese. There should be ½ cup of cheese remaining. Set this aside.

3) Cover with foil and bake for 30 minutes. The mixture should be bubbly and all the cheese melted. Remove from the oven. Sprinkle with the remaining cheese and add the chopped lettuce and salsa before serving. Serve immediately.

Makes 6 portions: 1 protein, 1 vegetable, 1 bread/starch, and 1 fat per serving.

BREAKFAST

Breakfast truly is an important meal for pregnant women. You need to "break the fast" you created while you slept. A good breakfast can include fruit or juice, protein from milk and cereal, lean meat such as Canadian bacon, peanut butter on toast, a scoop of cottage cheese, or even a dish of yogurt. Any of the dairy foods carry a good supply of calcium. Include enough bread, toast, bagels, or muffins to satisfy your appetite.

Wholesome Whole-Grain Muffins

⑥

I keep a batch of these muffins in the freezer and reheat them when I need a snack or a yummy breakfast treat. Because they are made with whole-wheat flour, oatmeal, and wheat germ, they are a good source of magnesium, vitamin E, and fiber. These are all nutrients that are essential to good health, especially while pregnant.

½ cup all-purpose flour
¾ cup whole-wheat flour
¼ cup wheat germ
1½ cup oatmeal
1 tsp. baking soda
1 tsp. baking powder
½ cup packed brown sugar
1 cup low-fat milk
2 tbsp. vegetable oil
2 eggs, beaten slightly
½ cup dark corn syrup
½ cup maple syrup

1) Lightly oil 18 muffin cups or line a muffin pan with paper liners. Preheat oven to 375°F.

2) Combine the flour, wheat germ, oatmeal, baking soda, baking powder, and brown sugar, and mix until blended.

3) Make a well in the center of the dry ingredients and add all remaining ingredients. With a wooden spoon, stir until combined.

4) Fill prepared muffin cups evenly with batter and bake for 18 minutes. Poke a toothpick into the center of a muffin and pull out smoothly. If it is clean, the muffins are ready.

Makes 18 muffins: 1 bread/starch per serving.

Breakfast Burrito

◎

Prepare these the night before and let them heat up while you get ready for work or get family members ready for the day.

4 oz. sharp cheddar cheese, sliced thin or grated
2 oz. ham, chopped
4 soft 6-inch flour tortillas
Aluminum foil

1) Sprinkle a quarter of the cheese on half of each tortilla, along with a quarter of the chopped ham. Roll each tortilla so the cheese and ham are rolled up tight. Place each tortilla on a single sheet of aluminum foil and wrap the tortillas so they are covered tightly. Keep refrigerated until ready to heat.

2) Place in a 350°F oven and heat for ten minutes or until cheese melts. Eat while hot.

Makes four portions: 1 bread/starch, 1 protein per serving.

Variation: Veggie Tortillas
Sauté one small chopped onion and one small chopped
green pepper in 1 teaspoon of vegetable oil for about one
minute, until soft and the onion is translucent. Prepare tortillas as described above and divide the cooked vegetables
equally over the tortillas. Wrap and heat as directed above.

Makes 4 portions: 1 vegetable and 1 bread/starch per serving.

Tortilla Pancakes
◎

Make these on weekends for a special treat. Keep some
individually wrapped and frozen, ready to heat as needed for
a quick snack.

4 soft flour tortillas
2 cups cottage cheese
1 tsp. honey
1 tsp. granulated sugar
⅛ tsp. ground cinnamon

1) Mix the cottage cheese, honey, sugar, and cinnamon in
a food processor or electric blender until smooth.

2) Spread ½ cup of the cheese mixture on one side of each
tortilla. Fold in half and fold again into quarters. Wrap in
aluminum foil and bake for 15 minutes or until cheese is
hot. Eat as a snack or serve on a plate with syrup or
fresh fruit.

Makes four portions: 2 bread/starch, ½ calcium per serving.

Overnight French Toast

◎

When I was pregnant, I looked for recipes I could put together the night before and cook in the oven while I got ready for work. I like this recipe even more now that my kids are school age and mornings are hectic.

> 3 large eggs
> 1 cup skim milk
> ¼ tsp. cinnamon
> Fresh nutmeg for garnish
> 8 slices of your favorite bread, sliced ½ inch thick

1) Lightly oil a flat casserole dish. Beat the eggs, milk, and cinnamon together until well blended. Arrange the bread in the casserole dish (the bread can overlap if necessary). If the layer of bread is more than an inch thick, add another 15 minutes to the cooking time.

2) Pour the egg mixture over the bread, making sure every piece of bread is moistened. Cover with foil and refrigerate over night.

3) Place the French toast in a cold oven and turn the oven onto 375°F. Cook for at least 30 minutes. It should be golden and puffy when done, with no runny egg spots. Top with fresh nutmeg and serve with syrup and fresh fruit.

Makes four portions: 2 bread/starch, ⅓ protein, 1 fat, and ¼ calcium per serving.

DESSERT

Dessert can be a wholesome addition to meals, but don't overdo it. Many women, knowing they need to eat more calories when pregnant, go overboard on desserts. It is true that you need an extra 300 calories per day when pregnant, but did you know that just one slice of birthday cake can provide that and some premium ice creams can carry 400 calories per cup? Think about your dessert choices and don't throw caution entirely to the wind. Try to choose a dessert that carries a wholesome food from one of the six food groups, such as a milk-based pudding, a whole-grain cookie, or something sweetened with fruit.

Oatmeal Chocolate Chip Bars

◎

When you are craving chocolate, prepare a batch of these easy-to-make bars. Besides the good-tasting chocolate, they carry wholesome oatmeal and not too much added fat.

½ cup sugar
½ cup brown sugar
¼ cup softened butter
2 eggs
¼ cup low-fat milk
½ cup applesauce
1 cup all-purpose flour
½ cup whole-wheat flour
½ teaspoon baking soda
¼ teaspoon ground nutmeg

3 cups rolled oats
1 cup chocolate chips

1) Preheat oven to 350°F. Lightly oil a 9-inch x 13-inch brownie pan. In a large bowl, cream the sugars and the butter together until well combined. Add eggs, milk, and applesauce and mix until smooth.

2) In a separate bowl combine the flour, baking soda, and oats. Stir into the egg mixture, along with the chocolate chips. Blend until all dry ingredients are moistened and the chips are distributed evenly.

3) With a large spoon spread the batter into the prepared pan so that it is evenly distributed.

4) Bake in the preheated oven about 20 to 22 minutes, until the top is lightly browned. Remove from the oven, cut into 40 squares while warm. Cool in the pan.

Makes 40 squares: 1 bread/starch per serving.

Good News Cookies

◎

Not all things that taste good are bad for us. These cookies are made with whole-wheat flour and are a delicious alternative to ordinary sugar cookies.

5 tbsp. butter
¾ cup sugar
1 egg
1 tsp. vanilla

2 tbsp. wheat germ
¼ cup low-fat milk
1½ cups whole-wheat flour
½ tsp. baking powder
½ tsp. baking soda
½ tsp. cinnamon
¼ tsp. grated nutmeg
2 tbsp. brown sugar (for sprinkling)

1) Preheat oven to 350°F. Cream butter and sugar together until soft and fluffy.

2) Beat in egg, vanilla, wheat germ, and milk. In a small bowl combine the flour, baking powder, baking soda, cinnamon, and nutmeg.

3) Stir egg mixture into the dry ingredients until well blended. Drop by tablespoons onto a lightly oiled cookie sheet, sprinkle with the brown sugar and bake for ten minutes, until lightly browned.

Makes two dozen cookies: 1 bread/starch and 1 fat per cookie.

Sweet Potato Pudding

⚭

Here is a dessert that carries protein from egg, calcium from milk, and vitamin A and fiber from the sweet potato. It's a delicious way to get nutrients.

3 cups grated sweet potato
2 cups evaporated skim milk
½ cup sugar
3 large eggs
1 tsp. cinnamon
½ tsp. ginger
½ tsp. nutmeg

1) Preheat oven to 350°F. Combine all ingredients until well blended.

2) Pour into a lightly buttered 6-cup baking dish. Cook for 40 minutes until lightly browned and firm, like a custard. Serve warm or cold.

Makes 6 ½-cup portions: ½ calcium and 1 vegetable per serving.

Chocolate Bread Pudding with Meringue

This is one of my all-time favorite desserts. It has a real old-fashion goodness to it, far superior to ready-made puddings available at the market.

2 oz. unsweetened chocolate
2 cups milk
½ cup brown sugar
2 large eggs, separated
1 tsp. pure vanilla extract
6 slices day-old bread (try a handcut whole wheat)
¼ cup granulated sugar

1) Preheat oven to 350°F. In a heavy saucepan combine the chocolate with the milk and cook about 3–5 minutes, stirring often to prevent burning, until chocolate melts.

2) In a separate bowl, combine the brown sugar with the egg yolks and mix well.

3) Stir ¼ cup of the chocolate milk mixture into the egg-yolk mixture until well blended. Return the entire mixture to the saucepan for about four minutes, stirring frequently to prevent lumps. Stir in vanilla.

4) Tear the bread into bite-size pieces and stir it into the chocolate mixture so it is well coated but not mashed. Pour into a lightly buttered casserole dish and bake for 30 minutes.

5) While the pudding bakes, beat the egg whites until frothy, add the sugar, and continue beating until stiff peaks form.

6) After the pudding has baked for 30 minutes, spread the meringue on top and bake an additional 5–6 minutes until just golden. Serve warm.

Makes four portions: ½ calcium, 1½ bread/starch per serving.

Indian Pudding
◎

Assemble this pudding when you're home on a cold rainy weekend. It takes a while to bake, and the aroma will give your home a warm, comforting smell.

½ cup yellow cornmeal
3 cups milk
⅓ cup molasses
½ tsp. ginger

1) Pour the milk into a large, heavy saucepan and cook on medium heat until it is almost to a boil.

2) Reduce heat to low and slowly stir in cornmeal, breaking up any lumps that may appear. Add molasses and ginger, stirring continuously until it starts to thicken, about 8 minutes.

3) Pour into a lightly buttered baking dish and bake at 300°F for two hours or until thick and lightly browned on top.

Makes six portions: ½ calcium and 1 bread/starch per serving.

It's a Wrap!

"Wraps" have become popular at restaurants and are easy to prepare at home too. Use a soft flour tortilla, pita bread (sliced in half to make two thin circles), or a flat round bread called Mountain Bread available in many supermarkets. Try the whole-wheat versions as well as the white.

Veggie Wrap

Purchase your favorite chopped vegetables from the supermarket salad bar (broccoli, mushrooms, peppers), wrap them in an 8-inch tortilla, sliced pita pocket, or a

circle of Mountain Bread, sprinkle with 1 to 2 ounces of your favorite grated cheese and bake, covered in foil at 350°F for ten minutes or until hot.
Makes one portion: 1 bread/starch, 1 vegetable, 1 calcium.

Sweet Tooth Wrap

Chop your favorite chocolate candy bar into bite size pieces, wrap in a soft flour tortilla and microwave for one minute until the chocolate melts.
Makes one portion: 1 bread/starch, 2 fats.

Cinnamon Wrap

Sprinkle a soft flour tortilla with cinnamon sugar and bake at 350°F until it bubbles and becomes golden in color.
Makes one portion: 1 bread/starch.

5

Special Problems, Special Answers

Pregnancy is not a medical problem. It is a natural process—part of life. A small number of women, however, will experience medical complications during pregnancy. Conditions such as iron deficiency anemia, pregnancy-induced hypertension, and gestational diabetes are not uncommon. For women who have always experienced good health, it can be hard to accept any of these diagnoses. If you are informed of a complication that can affect your pregnancy and the health of your baby, one of your first challenges as a responsible mother will be to do just what the doctor orders.

IRON DEFICIENCY ANEMIA

Iron deficiency anemia is the nutrition problem women are most likely to encounter while pregnant. It occurs because a substantial amount of iron is needed during pregnancy to make red blood cells. One estimate puts the frequency of iron deficiency anemia at 10 percent of all pregnancies. It is a condition more common among the poor, but it is by no means restricted to any one socioeconomic group. Any woman eating a marginal diet can be at risk.

It is important to recognize and treat iron deficiency anemia because low levels of serum ferritin are associated with an increased risk for low-birth-weight babies and pre-term delivery. It also causes fatigue and shortness of breath.

The doctor will screen for a preexisting iron deficiency at your very first prenatal visit. Any woman who is found to have very low serum ferritin and hemoglobin levels is presumed to have iron deficiency anemia. It is usually treated with 60 to 120 mg. of ferrous iron until the hemoglobin becomes normal, at which time the dose decreases to 30 mg. per day.

It may sound as though iron supplements are a simple and automatic solution to the problem, but iron absorption is a complicated process. It is estimated that the total "cost" of a single normal pregnancy is about 500 to 800 mg. of iron. Nearly 300 mg. of that iron is needed by your growing baby, and the remainder is required by you to meet your own demands. It is in the last trimester that the need for iron is at its greatest, and if the supply—or more appropriately, the absorption and utilization of iron—is not adequate, it is the mother, not the baby, who will develop the iron deficiency.

It is almost impossible for any pregnant woman to actually meet the RDA for iron from food sources alone. The RDA for iron is set at 30 mg. per day for pregnant women, and the typical American diet carries about 6 to 7 mg. of iron for every 1,000 calories of food. That means that a woman taking in 2,500 calories can expect to consume about 15 to 18 mg. of iron from food sources alone. To make matters more complicated, the usual rate of iron absorption is only 10 percent. Fortunately, though the RDA is set at 30 mg. of dietary iron, it is estimated that only 4 to 7 mg. of iron needs to be absorbed and put into circulation by the mother. Also, during pregnancy the body's ability to absorb iron becomes more efficient and the rate of absorption jumps from 10 to 30 percent. And of course the monthly blood loss of menstruation stops at the beginning of a pregnancy, which is particularly useful in preventing iron depletion in the first trimester.

So the question really is: How much iron does a mother have to actually eat in order to meet the iron demands created by pregnancy? The woman who obtains 15 mg. of iron from food and takes 30 mg. of iron as a supplement should absorb 30 percent of that total, or 13.5 mg. This is an amount that can meet the pregnant woman's need for iron.

On the other hand, women are advised not to overdo it with iron. Too much supplemental iron can cause stomach irritation and constipation, and it may interfere with the absorption of other minerals such as zinc. Don't be terribly surprised if your doctor asks you to skip the iron supplement altogether. A study published in *American Journal of Obstetrics and Gynecology* in 1995 compared the outcomes of 2,944 pregnant women who were randomly divided into two groups: one group received iron only if it was needed, and the other group was given iron as a preventive measure. There were no statistical differences between the two groups in either the health of the women or the outcomes of the pregnancies. The authors of the study state that routine iron supplementation does not seem to be necessary for all women.

To reduce your risk of iron deficiency anemia:

◎ Eat one food rich in iron at every meal. The best iron sources include beef, lamb, pork, poultry, fish.

⑨ Consume a food rich in vitamin C at every meal. Vitamin C can enhance iron absorption. Include any citrus fruit or juice, tomatoes.

⑨ Select iron-fortified grain and bakery products.

⑨ Limit tea consumption. Tea can interfere with iron.

⑨ Discuss the use of iron supplements with your doctor. Take iron supplements only if they are recommended by your health-care provider.

⑨ If your prenatal supplement carries iron, and most of them do, make sure your doctor is aware of this before you take additional iron supplements.

GESTATIONAL DIABETES

While iron deficiency anemia is the most common nutrition disorder of pregnancy, gestational diabetes is the most common medical disorder of pregnancy effecting 2–6 percent of all pregnancies, or 90,000 American women each year. The woman who develops gestational diabetes will have a blood sugar level (glucose level) that is higher than normal. The condition can be managed effectively with a good diet, exercise, and proper follow-up.

Gestational diabetes is usually diagnosed in the second half of pregnancy and, in most cases, disappears after the baby is born. However, women who have gestational diabetes are believed to run a greater risk of developing diabetes as they grow older. Babies born to mothers with uncontrolled gestational diabetes may be larger in size (increasing the risk of complications at delivery), more prone to jaundice, and have low blood sugars when born. Babies born to mothers who have this condition will have their blood sugar checked at birth to make sure it is not low.

Your doctor will screen for gestational diabetes between the 24th and 28th week of pregnancy. Women who are considered at high risk may be screened earlier. The risk for gestational diabetes increases with each of these factors: obesity (BMI greater than 29); age (over 30 years); a family history of diabetes; a complicated previous pregnancy or a previous case of gestational diabetes; high blood pressure; and sugar in the urine.

To screen for gestational diabetes, you will be asked to consume 50 grams of glucose, which is the equivalent of 10 to 12 teaspoons of sugar. Then your blood sugar will be tested after one hour to see how your body reacts to the sugar load. A glucose level below 140 mg. per deciliter (dl) is considered normal. If the level is greater you will be asked to return for a three-hour glucose tolerance test in which you will first have a fasting blood sugar drawn, followed by a drink carrying 100 grams of carbohydrate, and three blood tests at one-hour intervals.

To meet the diagnosis of gestational diabetes, two of the blood sugars in the three-hour glucose test must be abnormal. When only one blood test is abnormal, the diagnosis of "glucose intolerance" is made and conservative dietary therapy will be advised.

Normal blood sugar values for a three-hour glucose tolerance test

fasting: < 105 mg per dl

one hour: < 190 mg per dl

two hours: < 165 mg per dl

three hours: < 145 mg per dl

Once the diagnosis of gestational diabetes is made, diet therapy becomes the cornerstone of treatment. Excessive food intake is likely to increase blood-sugar levels, and women will be advised to eat a diet that is adequate but not excessive. I often tell people to keep their feelings of hunger (on a scale of 1 to 10) in the 5 to 6 range. This prevents over- and undereating. In the May, 1996, *American Family Physician,* Dr. Kenneth Weller suggests the following guidelines for keeping calorie intake within desired levels. Use these numbers as a starting point, but consult your own physician for individualized attention.

✆ Women below IBW can consume about 16 to 18 calories per pound of present weight.

✆ Women at normal weight can consume 13 to 14 calories per pound of present body weight.

✆ Women who are overweight can consume 11 calories per pound of present weight.

Using these calculations, the 5'8" woman who began her pregnancy at a weight of 140 pounds and now weighs approximately 150 pounds will be able to manage her gestational diabetes on approximately 2,025 calories per day. The food groups described in Chapter 3 are ideally suited for women with gestational diabetes, but always check with your doctor for individualized instruction.

Exercise is also important in controlling blood glucose levels. One study found that regular exercise combined with diet therapy was more effective in controlling gestational diabetes than just diet alone. Most women with gestational diabetes will be encouraged to exercise three to four days a week for 15 to 30 minutes. Walking and swimming are great activities for the pregnant woman. If you have not been active prior to your pregnancy, start slowly by exercising five to ten minutes per day and then increase to 30 minutes as you get stronger. Do not exercise too hard or get too hot, and don't let your pulse go above 140 to 160 beats per minute. If you become dizzy or have back pain, stop all activity. If you have uterine contractions or vaginal bleeding, call your doctor right away. Read in Chapter 6 about safe exercise guidelines during pregnancy.

Your doctor will ask you to get frequent blood tests throughout your pregnancy. A normal blood sugar is generally thought to be 105 mg./dl. when fasting and less than 120 mg./dl. two hours after a meal. If a blood sugar remains above normal despite a program of exercise and sensible eating, injections of insulin may be required. Approximately 10 to 15 percent of women with gestational diabetes will require insulin treatment. Insulin, a hormone that regulates blood-sugar levels, is normally made by the body but is either absent or ineffective in people who have diabetes. In most cases, when insulin is required the diet and exercise program is the same, but it becomes crucial that meals are not delayed or skipped. Such a situation can actually result in a low blood sugar, which can cause dizziness and shaking. It can be treated by drinking juice, milk, or regular soda but it is better to prevent the problem simply by eating on schedule.

Women who are diagnosed with gestational diabetes are at an increased risk for developing the disorder in subsequent pregnancies, and they have a 50 percent chance of developing type 2 or non-insulin-dependent diabetes within the next 20 years. Once your baby is born, a lifestyle that includes regular exercise, healthy eating, and maintaining your weight at a BMI below 26 will go a long way toward preventing the disease as you get older.

Consider breast-feeding your baby as a means to control gestational diabetes. In a study of over 809 women it was found that even a short period of breast-feeding had a positive effect on gestational diabetes. Though all the women in the study were similar in age and weight, only 4 percent of the women who were breast-feeding at the 4 to 12 week follow-up appointment met the criteria for diabetes, as compared to 9 percent of the nonbreast-feeding mothers. Some research suggests that breast-feeding alone may actually reduce or delay a woman's risk of subsequent diabetes.

To manage gestational diabetes:

◎ Eat three moderate-sized meals per day with small snacks between meals.

◎ Eat a balanced diet including all food groups.

◎ Avoid foods that carry a lot of refined sugars and starches, such as frosted cakes, cookies, candy, and soda.

◎ Make at least three of your servings from the bread/ starch group whole-grain choices.

◎ Review weight-gain goals with your doctor, and adjust your food intake to meet them.

◎ Exercise as recommended by your doctor.

◎ You can decrease your risk of developing type 2 diabetes later in life by remaining active, and by preventing significant weight gain with age.

HYPERTENSION

Preeclampsia (pronounced pre-ee-*clamp*-see-ah) or toxemia, is a very serious condition characterized by high blood pressure, protein in the urine, and excessive edema (fluid retention). It affects some 7 percent of pregnant women, usually in the second half of their pregnancy. First-time mothers have a higher incidence, and the risk increases if other members of the family such as a sister or mother experienced the condition while pregnant. Women carrying multiple babies, and women over 40 or under 20 years of age are believed to be at a greater risk as well.

A blood pressure above 140/90 is defined as hypertension, but remember, just because your blood pressure is elevated does not mean you have preeclampsia. Other symptoms, such as protein in the urine and swelling that doesn't go away, must be present too.

Fortunately, preeclampsia can be controlled with early diagnosis and careful medical management. Early detection is one reason that regular prenatal checkups are so important. Preeclamsia can be harmful to the baby because it can prevent the placenta from getting enough blood, which is the baby's only supply of food and oxygen. When the placenta is not well nourished, the growing baby may not reach an ideal birth weight and, in some cases, the mother can experience seizures.

To control preeclampsia the doctor will want to lower a mother's blood pressure, possibly with bed rest or the use of medications. In some cases hospitalization may be required.

Bed Rest and Eating Well

Complete bed rest may be ordered as a way to manage pregnancy-related medical conditions. Bed rest can soon become tedious and boring, though, and snacking as a means of curbing boredom can easily lead to excessive weight gain. Conversely, some women complain that they get depressed and lose interest in food, which also affects the quality of their diet.

Nutrition Tips for When the Doctor Orders Bed Rest:

- Drink plenty of fluids. Keep a pitcher of water on hand.

- Keep a small refrigerator or cooler near the bed stocked with nutritious foods.

- Use ready-to-eat foods like peeled carrots, ready-made salads, rotisserie chickens.

- Keep a supply of your favorite frozen dinners on hand.

- Keep fresh fruit on hand.

- Constipation can be a side effect of inactivity. Adequate fluid and fiber may help: eat three whole-grain foods from the starch group, two whole fruits, and three servings of vegetables daily.

- Eat enough, but not an excessive amount of, protein. Keep to a total of approximately 7 ounces of meat, fish, or chicken per day and three to four glasses of milk. These two food groups carry the greatest source of protein per serving.

- Avoid fried foods and fried snack foods.

☙ Ask family or friends to grocery shop for you, using a food list that is planned with the help of the serving recommendations on pages 74–81.

A salt restriction can be useful in controlling blood pressure when not pregnant, but the pregnant woman requires salt and the sodium it contains to keep up the flow of fluids in the body. For this reason, the doctor will encourage you to maintain your normal salt intake. In some cases, fluid restriction may be advised. Do not restrict fluids unless specifically told to do so by your medical provider.

Clinical trials have shown aspirin to have a favorable effect on the reduction of preeclampsia, and some physicians are recommending its daily use, but aspirin is not recommended as a routine course of preventive treatment for all pregnant women. Calcium has long been studied for its potential effect on high blood pressure. One study found that when healthy, first-time mothers took calcium supplements at recommended levels, they decreased their risk of short-term high blood pressure. Though transient high blood pressure is benign, it forces more scrutiny and monitoring of a healthy pregnancy. A healthful diet with reasonable weight gain can assist in controlling blood pressure, but preeclampsia is a medical condition that can deteriorate or change rapidly and it requires close attention.

To reduce your risk of high blood pressure:

☙ Sleep on your left side. This takes the weight off large blood vessels and increases urine flow.

☙ Maintain a normal sodium intake.

☉   Eat a diet adequate in protein.

☉   Eat a diet adequate in calcium.

☉   A rapid weight gain of more than five pounds per week can indicate unhealthy fluid retention. Call your doctor.

CHOLESTEROL AND FAT

During pregnancy it is not unusual for cholesterol levels to rise as much as 25 to 40 percent. This increase is the result of hormone changes, which cause lipid levels to rise during pregnancy, only to return to their normal state after birth. The National Cholesterol Education Program recommends that all healthy individuals eat a diet that contains 30 percent fat and 10 percent saturated fat. There are few, if any, studies that support a low-fat menu for pregnant women, but there are no specific fat recommendations either. The 30 percent guideline is probably a reasonable level for pregnant women.

It is important for women to eat adequate amounts of fat during pregnancy. Foods that carry polyunsaturated fats and essential fatty acids may actually be beneficial to the visual and psychomotor development of the growing baby. Foods that carry beneficial fat sources include lean meat and poultry, fish, wheat germ and whole-grain foods such as whole-wheat bread, and salad dressings made with vegetable or cooking oils. If you are informed of a high cholesterol level while pregnant, the same balanced eating guidelines described in Chapter 3 will still apply in the majority of cases. Months after the baby is born your doctor may ask you to repeat a blood cholesterol test. Breast-feeding mothers tend to have higher cholesterol levels as a result of the normal changes in lipid levels associated with lactation, so make sure your doctor knows you are still breast-feeding. Women requiring a low-fat menu, to treat gallbladder problems or familial hyperlipidemia, should receive individualized diet instruction with the help of a registered dietitian.

PHENYLKETONURIA

Phenylketonuria (PKU) is the most common of the inherited disorders collectively referred to as an inborn error of metabolism. Phenylketonuria occurs when a newborn cannot convert excess phenylalanine, an essential amino acid, into a harmless amino acid called tyrosine. When too much phenylalanine accumulates in the tissue of the brain, it will cause mental retardation.

PKU occurs in approximately one in 12,000 live births. To detect this potentially devastating condition, all babies are checked for PKU within 72 hours of birth. A baby found to have PKU will be started on a special diet to keep phenylalanine levels low. When dietary treatment is started within the first 12 days of life, intelligence is normal.

Aspartame: Is it safe?

Aspartame is an artificial sweetener synthesized from two amino acids (one of which is phenylalamine). Despite years of testing it remains controversial and a source of concern for pregnant women. In a May, 1995, issue of the journal *American Family Physician,* Dr. William Hueston states that "though pregnant women are often concerned about this product, there are no studies of adverse effects to mother or baby." He states that even "patients with phenylketonuria can consume large doses of aspartame (34 to 100 mg. per kg.) without a significant increase in their phenylalanine levels." Nevertheless, women with phenylketonuria should avoid aspartame just to be safe.

Since aspartame carries no nutrients and because women need extra calories while pregnant, there seems to be no need for the use of aspartame during pregnancy, except possibly for women with diabetes. However, even these women are likely to tolerate small amounts of real sugar. Ask your doctor for guidance on this issue. For the majority of pregnant women, even though scientific evidence is lacking, avoiding aspartame might give you one less thing to worry about.

Screening for and treatment of the condition has been so successful that babies born with PKU are now old enough to have babies themselves. It is estimated that 3,000 young American women of reproductive age have an abnormality in their phenylalanine metabolism. Women with PKU who have relaxed their metabolic control must plan their pregnancies and adjust their diets significantly before and during pregnancy.

SMOKING

It is estimated that a baby born to a mother who smoked more than one pack of cigarettes per day during her pregnancy will weigh 7 to 8 ounces less than if the mother had not smoked. In addition, smoking increases the mother's risk of miscarriage and preterm delivery. The chemicals in smoke reduce a mother's ability to carry oxygen via blood to her baby. Smoking also causes constriction of the blood vessels, decreasing blood flow further and interfering with the baby's ability to get nutrients.

Mothers who smoke may be robbing their baby of vitamin C, which is often low in the blood of heavy smokers. In addition, smokers tend to have lower levels of carotene (a form of vitamin A), vitamin B_{12}, and zinc. Because cigarettes suppress appetite they can interfere with a woman's ability to eat enough food. This is particularly significant for women who are having difficulty gaining all the weight they need.

Also consider the environment your baby will live in once born. A child who lives in a home with parents who smoke will have more upper respiratory infections than children who live in a smoke-free environment. Not only are there numerous health reasons to quit, but also consider the financial costs. A family that spends $1.50 a day on cigarettes is spending over $500 a year. Quit smoking and force yourself to put this money away and just imagine what you could spend it on.

There are unpublished reports referred to in the textbook *Modern Nutrition* that find nicotine patches can help break the nicotine addiction without having an adverse effect on mother or baby. If you can't quit, at least reduce your smoking to under five cigarettes per day, as this decreases the health risks.

Women who choose to quit must recognize the effect it can have on their weight even while pregnant. In one study, women who quit smoking while pregnant gained more weight than nonsmokers or women who continued to smoke. This weight gain may reflect an increase in plasma fluid volume which is lower in smokers and is probably the reason fetal growth improves when women quit. Research finds that at one year postpartum, former smokers retain more weight than nonsmokers or women who continue to smoke. While it is essential to quit smoking, it is also important to acknowledge the potential impact it can have on your weight.

If you smoke:

◎ Inform your doctor about your smoking habits. Ask for advice on quitting.

◎ When you do quit, start a gentle exercise program to prevent weight retention.

◎ If you are a heavy smoker, be sure to take a multivitamin as described in Chapter 1.

◎ If you can't completely quit, at least cut down while you are pregnant.

OTHER HARMFUL SUBSTANCES

Alcohol

Alcohol has the unique distinction of being both a liquid food, because it contains calories, and a drug. As a drug it can affect behavior, causing a loosening of inhibitions and an impairment of judgment. Since 1973 the deleterious effects of heavy alcohol use on fetal development have been studied. Babies born to heavy drinkers go on to display a range of symptoms referred to as fetal alcohol syndrome, which has a permanent effect on growth, development, and intelligence.

Approximately 2 to 3 percent of pregnant women are chronic drinkers. Another 5 percent of pregnant women have a drink every day, and 3 percent have a drink three times per week. Half of all women have an occasional drink while pregnant. Because of the effect alcohol can have on the baby, women are advised simply *not to drink while pregnant.*

◎ Discuss the use of alcohol with your doctor.

◎ If you find it difficult to give up, consult a therapist trained in substance abuse.

Caffeine

Seventy-four percent of American women consume 100 to 150 mg. of caffeine daily from coffee, tea, cola drinks, and chocolate. Caffeine is a central nervous system stimulant and during pregnancy it has an extended half-life. For years there has been a question about its effect on pregnancy. Some studies have suggested that caffeine is a risk factor for reduced birth weight and that it increases the risk of birth defects and miscarriage. Studies of women who consumed more than 300 mg. of caffeine per day do have a greater risk for delivering smaller babies, but the research has not been able to determine whether it is the caffeine or other lifestyle factors that cause the lower birth weights.

Caffeine Content of Selected Foods

12 oz. cola	37 mg.
6 oz. coffee*	103 mg.
6 oz. brewed tea	36 mg.
1 oz. chocolate candy	13 mg.
1 chocolate fudge pop	3 mg.
8 oz. chocolate milk	8 mg.
6 oz. hot chocolate from mix	4 mg.

*A small take-out coffee is 10 to 12 oz., a large is 16 oz.

We do know that mothers who are heavy caffeine consumers could cause caffeine withdrawal in their newborns, which will cause feeding difficulties, excessive crying, poor sleep, and irritability. Because of the potential effect on the baby, pregnant mothers should keep their caffeine consumption moderate, that is, less than 300 mg. or two cups of coffee per day. Keep in mind that other beverages can carry caffeine too.

Drugs

Just don't do it. All drugs reach an equilibrium between the mother's blood and the baby's within 30 minutes of ingestion or injection. Crack cocaine and cocaine are probably the most severe in their effect on the baby. Cocaine readily crosses the placenta, and women who use these drugs severely compromise the health of their babies.

Marijuana is probably perceived as a less risky drug, which explains why 10 to 27 percent of pregnant women admit to using marijuana while pregnant. Marijuana's effects on the developing fetus are similar to those of cigarettes. It interferes with the blood's ability to carry oxygen and decreases blood flow to the uterus, interfering with nutrient delivery. Like alcohol, it also has the ability to affect a woman's judgment, potentially causing her to participate in other high-risk behavior.

Don't forget about the potential side effects of over-the-counter drugs or prescription medicines. Before taking any medication discuss it carefully with the doctor and the pharmacy. Even a product that is safe and used routinely at other times in your life may be dangerous when you are pregnant.

6

Mommies in Motion

The physically fit pregnant woman is an image promoted on book covers and in magazine pictures. She is always smiling and appears surprisingly light on her feet, almost springing off the pavement with every step. Some women do bounce into their doctor's office, even in the last trimester, but many women find that the shift in their center of gravity, together with the extra weight they carry, slows them down, making them a bit less perky even if they are physically fit. There is no reason for a healthy woman to stop being active while pregnant but at the same time it is important to remember that pregnancy brings physical changes that affect how a woman moves, breathes, and bends.

Exercise has many benefits, but there is no evidence that it improves the health of your unborn baby. If you were not very active before becoming pregnant, now is not the time to start a vigorous plan. On the other hand, pregnancy is not the time to stop being active. Exercise and physical activity can help your sense of well-being by reducing pregnancy-related symptoms such as backache, constipation, bloating, and fatigue. It can also improve your emotional state of mind. So don't stop being active, but don't go overboard either. Just be aware that while you are pregnant things really are different.

One of the most profound changes you will experience while pregnant is a shift in your center of gravity. As you progress in your pregnancy the uterus enlarges, as do your breasts, and this shifts your weight to affect your sense of balance. A woman in her last trimester may find rocky paths difficult, her bowling arm to be unreliable, and bike-riding impossible.

Another change that can affect your level of activity is in your joints, which loosen during pregnancy, increasing your risk of sprains or falls. Exercises such as full sit-ups and double leg raises may strain the back, and straight-leg toe touches are discouraged due to softened connective tissue between muscles and joints. Pregnant women are also advised to avoid bouncy, jerky forms of exercise such as regular aerobics.

As your pregnancy progresses, your heart must work harder to pump the increased volume of blood in your body. You will find you reach your target heart rate sooner. According to the American College of Obstetricians and Gynecologists, pregnant women should not exceed 140 heartbeats per minute while exercising, and normally sedentary women should not engage in more than 15 to 20 minutes of strenuous exercise while pregnant.

Warning: Stop activity if any of these symptoms occur:

Pain

Dizziness

Shortness of breath

Feeling faint

Vaginal bleeding

Rapid heart rate while resting

Difficulty walking

Uterine contractions

No fetal movements

Body position affects exercise, too. If you lie on your back to exercise, be aware that the weight of your enlarged uterus can obstruct blood flow in the large veins that return blood to the heart. The resulting faintness and discomfort are known as *supine hypotensive syndrome*, which is remedied when you turn onto your side to allow blood flow to return to normal.

Most pregnant women experience a shortness of breath faster than usual when they are active. For some women it can be hard to keep up with the oxygen demands created by pregnancy. Also, as the uterus enlarges, it restricts the lungs and diaphragm, making the problem even more bothersome.

Pregnant women often joke about how their need for coats and sweaters diminishes even in winter. The increase in heat production caused by pregnancy is real, and it can be significant in the exercising woman. Studies suggest that even moderate exercise can increase body-core temperature. Fit women are believed to regulate their body temperatures better than the less active woman. However, since animal studies suggest that high body temperatures might be harmful to a developing baby, particularly early on in pregnancy, it is prudent for women to prevent becoming overheated through exertion. The American College of Obstetricians and Gynecologists suggests that active women should check body temperature either rectally or under the arm after an exercise routine. The temperature reading should be less than 101°F. Since dehydration can increase body temperature, drink plenty of fluids and avoid prolonged strenuous exercise in hot weather.

Women at risk for preterm labor may add to that risk if they exert themselves more than they should. Norepinephrine, a hormone that is increased by activity, also plays a significant role during labor, when it stimulates uterine contractions. Any woman at risk for premature labor must discuss the role of exercise with her doctor.

WHAT TO EXPECT

Most women find that they slow down while pregnant and many women stop exercising by the third trimester. Women often find that they become tired faster and find exercise to be less pleasurable in the last trimester because of the physical changes. Women who swim or use a stationary bike to keep active may find they can continue these activities longer through their pregnancy than they can jogging or walking.

All women need to have a frank discussion with their doctors about exercise during pregnancy. Tell your doctor exactly what your prepregnancy activities were. Women who have high blood pressure, who are underweight, or who are at risk for premature delivery need expert individual counseling about the amount and type of activity that is best for them.

When Not to Exercise

The American College of Obstetricians and Gynecologists has identified the following conditions as reasons to avoid exercise during pregnancy:

⑨ Pregnancy-induced hypertension

⑨ Premature rupture of membranes

⑨ Preterm labor during a prior or current pregnancy or both

⑨ Incompetent/cervix/cerclage

⑨ Persistent second- or third-trimester bleeding

⑨ Intrauterine growth retardation

⑨ Women with medical conditions including chronic hypertension or active thyroid, cardiac, vascular or pulmonary disease should determine with the help of their doctor if an exercise program is appropriate for them while pregnant.

The American College of Obstetricians and Gynecologists has written the following general recommendations to educate women about exercising while pregnant.

1) During pregnancy, women can continue mild to moderate exercise routines. Regular exercise, three times per week, is preferable to intermittent exercise.

2) Women should avoid exercises in the supine position or activities that require prolonged periods of motionlessness.

3) Women have decreased oxygen available to them when pregnant and should modify the intensity of their workouts accordingly. Women should stop exercising when they become fatigued. Do not continue exertion until you reach exhaustion.

4) Avoid any exercise that could result in injury due to loss of balance. Avoid any activity that risks even mild abdominal trauma.

5) Eat appropriately, including snacks between meals to keep yourself well fueled.

6) During exercise, particularly in the first trimester, help your body to dissipate heat by drinking plenty of fluids, wearing appropriate clothing, and exercising in a healthy environment.

7) After delivery, many of the changes produced by pregnancy continue for 4–6 weeks postpartum, so resume your prepregnancy activities slowly.

ACTIVITIES DURING PREGNANCY

Walking: Walking is the easiest of activities to include in your life, and it is usually a good activity even when you are pregnant. As your pregnancy progresses, be careful and try to walk on level paths.

Swimming: Swimming can be continued safely while you are pregnant. However, do not dive later in pregnancy, and do not scuba dive while pregnant.

Jogging: In general, women who jogged before they became pregnant can continue a moderate jogging program while pregnant. Discuss the duration of your jogging program with your doctor. Do not become overheated, and be sure to keep well hydrated.

Tennis: Balance and sudden stops can become problematic later in pregnancy. Consider playing doubles instead of singles (to keep exertion down).

Skiing: Consider a switch to cross-country skiing over downhill skiing. Cross-country skiing can be less dangerous if you ski slowly and select level trails. Hard falls can be serious while pregnant. High-altitude skiing is discouraged because of decreased oxygen.

Water skiing: This sport is discouraged because a fall at high speed can be dangerous to the baby.

Note that aerobics classes designed for the nonpregnant women are likely to involve jerky, jumpy movements. These classes are not recommended during pregnancy.

EXERCISE AND FOOD

In theory, women require an additional 300 calories daily while pregnant, but women who regularly exercise may need more than that. In addition to extra calories, a woman may need to eat more carbohydrates. While pregnant, women have lower fasting blood-sugar levels and use carbohydrates at a greater rate than when they are not pregnant.

Some pregnant women may be at greater risk for hypoglycemia or low blood sugar. Hypoglycemia is characterized by lightheadedness, shakiness, and weakness. Women who experience this can prevent it by eating regular meals, snacking between meals, and eating carbohydrates before and during prolonged activity. Try snacking on foods from the fruit or starch group before and during an activity.

Some women need to add protein to their snack regime. Foods such as a glass of milk, a cup of yogurt, a slice or two of cheese, or a tablespoon of peanut butter on top of a cracker contain protein as well as carbohydrate. If low-blood-sugar symptoms continue, discuss this with your doctor.

AFTER THE BABY

One of the greatest adjustments you will have to make, once you have a baby in tow, is finding the time for the activities you enjoy. First of all, allow yourself at least four to six weeks to adjust after the birth. If you had a cesarean birth talk to your doctor about when to start exercise. Four to six weeks is the usual recommendation. Read more about exercising after the baby is born in the next chapter.

7

After the Baby

After all these months the baby is finally here and now you are ready to reclaim your old self. The old you is still there, just a bit repressed by your new role as mother. Don't be at all surprised if you are not constantly elated in this new role. Most of us underestimate the demands motherhood bring. Some women experience mild, even severe, depression following delivery.

For most women, returning to their prepregnancy weight is a major goal, part of the recapture of the old self. The first four to six weeks after delivery are a time of adjustment. Get the rest you need, and adjust to the rhythm of the new family you have created. Eat sensibly, taking the time to eat three meals and appropriate snacks. Let friends and family help you with meals. Keep ready-to-eat foods on hand, so you don't have to spend a lot of time on food preparation.

Though most women want to return to their prepregnancy weight right away, it does not usually happen immediately, and you will have no control over some aspects of your weight. In the first four days after birth many women actually gain weight, but weight loss usually begins by the fifth day. If you had medical conditions such as hypertension or preeclampsia during pregnancy, weight loss may be above average because of increased fluid losses. Breast-feeding mothers may find they lose weight consistently in the first few weeks, only to slow to one to two pounds per month later on.

It is normal for women to lose weight in the four to six months after delivery, but not all women do. Lifestyle changes that accompany motherhood can lead women to eat foods that are less than ideal. Preparing healthful, low-calorie meals is often delayed as the baby is tended to. Many women who have quit full-time work will find snacking to be a problem. It is also more difficult to arrange exercise time. Also, if you stopped smoking while you were pregnant, it will probably be harder for you to lose weight than for other women who never smoked. Do not start smoking again. It will be just as hard to quit the next time and secondary smoke is harmful to your baby.

You should have a postpartum doctor's visit four to six weeks after delivery. This is usually a great time to monitor weight. The doctor's office scales are often more objective because they have the weight recorded from the first prenatal visit. Studies show that many women underestimate their pre-conception weight, adding to the notion that pregnancy causes permanent weight gain. Ask for guidance about reasonable weight-loss goals. A weight loss of 13 ounces to 1 pound per week is recommended. This is also the time to talk about exercise. Women who are overweight, or who have high blood pressure, a history of chest pains, or shortness of breath should get their doctor's permission before starting an exercise program. Exercise is encouraged for all women as part of a comprehensive fitness program.

GOOD NUTRITION AFTER DELIVERY

It is possible that your stores of calcium, vitamin B_6, and folate need to be replenished. This can be accomplished by eating a balanced diet and eating the recommended servings of milk, protein, and vegetables, particularly green leafy ones. Read more about sources of these nutrients in Chapter 1. If you are planning another pregnancy within the next eighteen months it will be important for your body to restock these vital nutrients, especially folic acid. The mother who is well nourished between pregnancies is more likely to have a healthier pregnancy and larger baby.

Nutrition Before Conception

If you plan on becoming pregnant within the next 12 to 18 months keep these tips in mind:

ॐ Get the calcium you need. Adequate calcium is good for your bones and eating adequate amounts may prevent pregnancy complications, too.

ॐ Keep caffeine intake low. High caffeine intake has been known to delay conception. Limit your coffee to less than two cups per day.

ॐ Take 400 mcg. of supplemental folic acid to reduce your baby's risk of neural tube defects.

ॐ If you are underweight, try to eat enough to bring you above a BMI of 20.

ॐ If you are overweight, eat a healthful diet and walk every day, unless there is a medical reason preventing it.

ॐ Do not take large doses of supplemental vitamin A.

Women who have had twins or who are at risk for eating inadequately because of medical or emotional problems are advised to continue low doses of vitamin-mineral supplements. Women who had gestational diabetes, hypertension, or low iron levels should have these conditions evaluated at the first postpartum visit. If you had low iron levels while pregnant you are likely to find the problem corrected. Hematocrit and hemoglobin blood levels usually rise after delivery as blood volume contracts and red blood cells are released and made available for use in hemoglobin.

The Postpartum Diet

The woman who uses the following eating plan as a guide and eats to appetite will keep herself well nourished and gradually reduce her weight. These food groups add up to a total calorie intake in the 1,700 to 2,200 calorie range. Remember that pregnancy is really an 18-month experience because eating well after the baby is born is important, too. What you eat will effect your mood, energy levels, and sense of well-being.

For good postpartum nutrition, eat the following servings from each food group every day:

Calcium-rich	2–4 servings
Protein-rich	2 small servings, or 6–7 oz.
Bread/starch	7–9 servings
Vegetable	2–4 servings
Fruit	3–5 servings
Fat	5 servings

BREAST-FEEDING, NUTRITION AND WEIGHT LOSS

Weight loss in the first month postpartum can be erratic. After the first month, expect to lose one to two pounds a month and do not exceed a weight loss above four and a half pounds. When weight loss is too fast it indicates a low calorie intake. A mother who does not eat enough food may slow her baby's own rate of weight gain. Remember too, that as long as you are nursing your baby, your breasts, which are now much larger in size, will add at least two to three pounds to the scale and possibly more.

Breast-feeding mothers need to eat an additional 500 calories more per day than nonnursing mothers. These calories are needed for milk production, and the extra food carries additional nutrients to make breast milk. The nutrients that are most important to breast-feeding women are calcium, zinc, magnesium, vitamin B_6, and folic acid. It is recommended that breast-feeding mothers eat in the range of 2,200 to 2,700 calories. In theory, women need 2,700 calories per day while nursing. That number is determined by adding 500 calories to the 2,200 calories women need for weight maintenance. Food surveys conducted on breast-feeding mothers have shown that women can be in good health and have a well-nourished baby even when eating well below this 2,700 calorie level. Some women may need all those 2,700 calories but others may need far fewer. Activity, body height, and size are all factors that determine caloric needs.

To insure good nutrition, eat at least 1,800 calories and aim to lose one to two pounds per month. If your weight loss is faster than this or above four and a half pounds per month you are not eating enough food and you must increase your total food intake.

I'M NOT LOSING ANYMORE

If weight loss stops short of your desires you may need to examine both your eating and your exercise routine. Develop a fitness plan, not just a weight-loss plan. A fitness plan will serve you and your baby by keeping you well nourished and energized and by setting an example for your child. You are his first teacher and what you eat effects him in ways that are immeasurable. The first time you nurse or bottlefeed your baby you teach your child his first lesson about food and transmit your own ideas and attitudes about food and feeding. These messages will become even more profound as you introduce solids and as your baby sees how and what you eat.

Your Eating Plan

First decide on a healthy menu for yourself by starting with the food group serving suggestions discussed above. If you need more structure, return to Chapter 3 and find the method for determining calorie calculations. Multiply your ideal body weight by the activity number that fits your activity level. The resulting number is the number of calories you need to maintain your present weight.

In theory, to lose one pound per week, subtract 500 calories from this maintenance number. For example a sedentary mom who is 5'8" tall requires 1,820 calories to maintain an ideal body weight of 140 pounds. If she now weighs 160 pounds and wants to reduce to a weight of 140 pounds she should reduce her food intake by 500 calories daily to a level of 1,320. If she adheres to a 1,320-calorie menu for the next 20 weeks and loses one pound per week she will reach her target weight of 140 pounds. Once she reaches that level she should return to the 1,820 level to maintain it.

Use these calculations simply as guidelines. If subtracting 500 calories puts you below 1200 calories then that number is too low. Women are never advised to go below 1200 calories because at this level it becomes difficult to eat enough food to get all the nutrition you need. Once you know your calorie goal, select the number of food servings that you need to eat daily in order to meet it.

CALORIE CHART

	Calcium	Protein	Bread/ starch	Vegetable	Fruit	Fat
1,200	2	2	6	3	2	2
1,300	2	2	6	3	3	2
1,400	2	2	6	3	3	3
1,500	2	2	6	3	3	3
1,600	2	2	7	3	3	3
1,700	2	2–3	8	3	3	3

Your Exercise Plan

The next essential part of a fitness plan is exercise. Exercise can tone muscles and improve your cardiovascular system and sense of well-being. The activity I recommend most is walking. It is safe, inexpensive, and very enjoyable, and best of all you can do it for life. Walking with baby in a stroller can be a great way for you to get exercise, and the baby can get fresh air, too. Find a backpack or front pack that is comfortable for you and that supports the baby properly. You may also want to swap exercise time with another mom. You take her child for 20 minutes and she takes yours the next day. Such an arrangement also has the advantage of making a schedule you have to stick to.

To get the most out of a walking program you will want to stretch beforehand. If you feel any strains or pains you've gone too far. To stretch your hamstring muscles, stand about 12 to 18 inches away from the wall. Place your palms on the wall and keep your feet flat on the floor. You should feel a gentle pull. Some of the best stretches can be found in a book by Bob Anderson simply called *Stretching* (listed in Recommended Reading on page 182).

Before starting a walking program, get your doctor's approval and determine your target heart rate by consulting the chart below. To determine your heart rate, count your pulse immediately after exercising. Do this by feeling for the blood vessel that runs along your neck, under your jaw. You can also count the pulse on your wrist. After exercising, count your pulse for ten seconds and multiply it by 6. This is your heart rate per minute. Compare this number to the recommended heart rate for your age. When you are just starting out keep in the low range for your age. Once you become fit you can exercise to within the higher range.

TARGET HEART RATE FOR NONPREGNANT WOMEN

Age (years)	Target Heart Rate (beats per minute)	Average Maximum Heart Rate (beats per minute)
20	120–160	200
25	117–156	195
30	114–152	190
35	111–148	185
40	108–144	180
45	105–140	175
50	102–136	170
55	99–132	165
60	96–128	160
65	93–124	155
70	90–120	150

Source: (U.S. Department of Health and Human Services; Public Health Service; National Institutes of Health; National Heart, Lung, and Blood Institute. *Exercise and Your Heart.* NIH Publication No. 81–1677. U.S. Government Printing Office: Washington, DC, 1981).

To find your target heart rate, look for the age category closest to your age and read the line across. For example, if you are 43, the closest age on the chart is 45; the target heart rate is 105–140 beats per minute. Your maximum heart rate is usually 220 minus your age. Your target heart rate is 60–80 percent of the maximum. These figures are averages to be used as general guidelines and *do not apply to pregnant women.*

If you were inactive before pregnancy, try to find a way to

add exercise to your life now. Keeping active can reduce your risk of serious illness later in life including heart disease, cancer, osteoporosis, and obesity. Exercise has the added plus of influencing your child, too. Children who are raised by active parents are more likely to be active themselves.

General postpartum guidelines:

- Find an exercise you like and do it three times per week.

- Wear a good sports bra. If you are nursing you may need extra support; wear the nursing bra and slip a running bra over it.

- Beware of including baby in all your activities. Baby Joggers are great but a collision with another runner, animals, bikes, or even cars is obviously a danger. Travel on sidewalks and where the risk of collision is not great.

- Do not jog with baby in a backpack. The jarring motion can shake a baby's head, possibly causing damage. The same risk is present when taking a baby on a bike over very bumpy terrain. Baby Joggers are designed for smooth riding and they are the only way to include baby in your jogging routine.

- In cold weather, a baby in a Baby Jogger or carrier may become too cold.

- Sunburn and dehydration can occur when hiking or traveling with baby in hot weather. Use sunblock and umbrellas to protect tender skin from the sun.

- Put a safety helmet on your baby when jogging in a stroller and use the safety strap.

- Do not overexert yourself when jogging with baby.

How Often Should I Check My Weight?

Don't check your weight often. You have no control over the scale. Instead ask yourself: Am I exercising regularly (three to seven times per week)? Am I eating a healthful diet? These are the factors you can control. If you answer yes to these questions your body will reach the body weight that is right for your height and age. The scale only seems to frustrate women and enforce the notion of restrictive, unhealthy eating.

Some new mothers can lose the weight almost effortlessly, but not everyone does. The best strategy is a healthy diet combined with a consistent exercise program that you enjoy. Take things slowly and don't get frustrated. If you find yourself starting a fitness plan and then stopping, don't give up. Just start again. In my years as a dietitian (more than 20) I have found that people often need to start and restart their fitness programs. While you may not be perfect, it is better to set a positive goal and meet it at least some of the time then to set no goal at all.

CLOSING THOUGHTS

While you are pregnant take care of yourself. Do everything you need to do to make your pregnancy as healthy as it can be, then relax and enjoy the experience. Your body will do all the work and worrying will not make the baby any healthier. If there is a special restaurant you'd like to go to or trip you want to take, indulge yourself and find the time to do it before the baby arrives. Few women have much time after the baby is born. This means less time to exercise, to plan meals, or even to relax and read a book. Many mothers tell me the evening hours, when the baby (or babies) are sleeping, is the time they like to call their own, a time to have a special snack, a time to simply be alone. These are lifestyle changes that come with being a mother. They are common and they are temporary.

Parenting is worth all the effort it requires. It connects you to the world in a way that makes life richer. Most women will be healthier if they do not get completely lost in the role of mothering. Take care of yourself. Find time to eat well, exercise when you can, play with the baby, laugh with those you love, pursue your interests. You will never get all the laundry done or your house as clean as you might like it. These chores will always be there, but your babies won't be. They grow up, and so do we.

Resources

The following are additional sources of information about nutrition and pregnancy.

ORGANIZATIONS

American Academy of Pediatrics
141 Northwest Point Road
P.O. Box 927
Elk Grove Village, IL 60007

American College of Obstetricians and Gynecologists
409 12th Street, S.W.
Washington, DC 20024-2188

American Dietetic Association
216 W. Jackson Boulevard, Suite 800
Chicago, IL 60606-6995
1-800-877-1600

La Leche League International
P.O. Box 1209
Franklin Park, IL 60131
708-455-7730 or 1-800-LALECHE

RECOMMENDED READING

I have found the following books about health, cooking, and childrearing to be very useful and pertinent today, even though some were published in the 1980s. I recommend them for your own further reading.

Anderson, Bob, *Stretching*. Shelter Publications, Volinas, California, 1980.

Brody, Jane, *Jane Brody's Nutrition Book: A Lifetime Guide to Good Eating for Better Health and Weight Control*. W. W. Norton & Co., Inc., New York, 1985.

Leach, Penelope, *Your Baby and Child*. Rev. ed. Alfred A. Knopf, New York, 1989.

Rombauer, Irma S. *The All New All Purpose Joy of Cooking*. Scribner, New York, 1997.

Sater, Ellyn, R.D. *Child of Mine: Feeding with Love and Good Sense*. Bull Publishing Co., Menlo Park, CA, 1986.

White, Burton L. *The First Three Years of Life*. Prentice Hall, Inc., Englewood Cliffs, N.J., 1985.

Selected Bibliography

Much of the nutrition and health information for this book was based on material from the following resources. In addition to these references, specific articles that may of interest to the reader are also listed here under the chapter that discusses the particular topic.

Institute of Medicine, Subcommittee on Nutritional Status and Weight Gain During Pregnancy, *Nutrition During Pregnancy*, National Academy Press, Washington, D.C., 1990.

Ludewig, Patricia Wieland, *Essentials of Maternal-Newborn Nursing*. 3rd ed. Addison-Wesley Nursing, Redwood City, Calif., 1994

Shils, Maurice E., M.D. *Modern Nutrition in Health and Disease*. 8th ed., Lea & Febinger, Philadelphia, Pa., 1994.

Introduction

Abraham, S. "Attitudes to Body Weight Gain and Eating Behavior in Pregnancy." *Journal of Psychosomatic Obstetrics and Gynecology* December 15(4):189–195, 1994.

Fahy, Thomas A. "The Clinical Significance of Eating Disorders in Obstetrics." *British Journal of Obstetrics and Gynaecology* August 100:708–710, 1993.

Manson, JoAnn, et al. "A Prospective Study of Obesity and Risk of Coronary Heart Disease in Women." *New England Journal of Medicine* March 29 322:882–889, 1990.

Chapter 1

Abrams, B. "Factors Associated with the Pattern of Maternal Weight Gain During Pregnancy." *Obstetrics and Gynecology* 86:170–176, 1995.

Abrams, B. "Weight Gain and Energy Intake During Pregnancy." *Clinical Obstetrics and Gynecology* September 37(3):515–527, 1994.

Cogswell, M.E. "Gestational Weight Gain Among Average-weight and Overweight Women—What is Excessive?" *American Journal of Obstetrics and Gynecology* February 172:705–712, 1995.

Davies, K. "Body Image and Dieting in Pregnancy." *Journal of Psychosomatic Research* 38(8):787–799, 1994.

Dawes, M. G. "Patterns of Maternal Weight Gain in Pregnancy" *British Journal of Obstetrics and Gynaecology* 98(2):195–201, 1991 Feb.

Dewey, K. "Effects of Dieting and Physical Activity on Pregnancy and Lactation." *American Journal of Clinical Nutrition* 59(suppl.):446S–453S, 1994.

Ekblad, U. "Maternal Weight, Weight Gain During Pregnancy and Pregnant Outcome." *International Journal of Gynecology and Obstetrics* December 39(4):277–283, 1992.

Fahy, T. A. "The Clinical Significance of Eating Disorders in Obstetrics." *British Journal of Obstetrics and Gynecology* August 100:708–710, 1993.

Fahy, T. A. "Eating Disorders in Pregnancy." *Psychological Medicine* 21:577–580, 1991.

Franko, D. L. "Pregnancy and Eating Disorders: A Review and Clinical Implications." *International Journal of Eating Disorders* 13(1):41–48, 1993.

Keppel, K. "Pregnancy-Related Weight Gain and Retention: Implications of the 1990 Institute of Medicine's Guidelines." *American Journal of Public Health* 83:1100–1103, 1993.

Lederman, S. A. "The Effect of Pregnancy Weight Gain on Later Obesity." *Obstetrics and Gynecology* 82:148–155, 1993.

Williamson, D. F. "A Prospective Study of Childbearing and 10-year Weight Gain in U.S. White Women 25 to 45 Years of Age." *International Journal of Obesity: Related Metabolic Disorders* August 18(8):561–569, 1994.

Chapter 2

American College of Obstetricians and Gynecologists Committee Opinion "Folic Acid for the Prevention of Recurrent Neural Tube Defects." *AGOG Technical Bulletin*, March 120:1–3, 1993.

Clark, P. M. "Weight Gain in Pregnancy, Triceps Skinfold Thickness and Blood Pressure in Offspring." *Obstetrics and Gynecology* January 91(1):103–107, 1998.

Dahle, L. O. "The Effect of Oral Magnesium Substitution on Pregnancy-Induced Leg Cramps." *American Journal of Obstetrics and Gynecology* 173:175–180, 1995.

Fisher, M. "Nutrition Evaluation of Published Weight Reducing Diets." *Journal of the American Dietetic Association* April 85:450–454, 1985.

Kolasa, K. "Nutrition During Pregnancy." *American Family Physician* July 56(1):205–212, 1997.

Kousen, M. "Treatment of Nausea and Vomiting in Pregnancy." *American Family Physician* November 15:1279–1284, 1993.

"Long-term Effects of Iron Supplements During Pregnancy" (review). *American Family Physician* November 1, 52(6):1895–1896, 1995.

"Nausea and Vomiting During Pregnancy" (review). *American Family Physician,* October, 48(5):930, 1993.

Yates, A. A. "Dietary Reference Intakes: The New Basis for Recommendations for Calcium and Related Nutrients, B Vitamins, and Choline." *Journal of the American Dietetic Association.* June 98:669–709, 1998.

Chapter 3

King, J. "Energy Metabolism During Pregnancy: Influence of Maternal Energy Status." *American Journal of Clinical Nutrition* 59(suppl.):439S–445S, 1994.

Chapter 5

"Benefits of Lactation in Gestational Diabetes" (review). *American Family Physician* 49(3):666–671, 1994.

Hachey, D. "Benefits and Risk of Modifying Maternal Fat Intake in Pregnancy and Lactation." *American Journal of Clinical Nutrition* 59(suppl.):454S–464S, 1994.

Hemminki, E. "Long-term Follow-up of Mothers and Their Infants in a Randomized Trial on Iron Prophylaxis during Pregnancy." *American Journal of Obstetrics and Gynecology* July 173(1):205–209, 1995.

Hueston, W. J. "Common Questions Patients Ask During Pregnancy." *American Family Physician* May :1465–1470, 1995.

"Nutrition During Pregnancy." American College of Obstetricians and Gynecologists *(ACOG) Technical Bulletin* April 179:1–7, 1993.

Waisbren, S. "Psychosocial Factors in Maternal Phenylketonuria: Women's Adherence to Medical Recommendations." *American Journal of Public Health* 85:1636–1641, 1995.

Weller, K. "Diagnosis and Management of Gestational Diabetes." *American Family Physician* May 1 53(6):2053–2057, 1996.

Zamorski, M. "Preeclampsia and Hypertensive Disorders of Pregnancy." *American Family Physician* April 53(5): 1595–1604, 1996.

Chapters 6 and 7

"Exercise During Pregnancy and the Postpartum Period." *ACOG Technical Bulletin* February 189:1–5, 1994.

"Women and Exercise." *ACOG Technical Bulletin* October 173:1–9, 1992.

Index